Hanane BENALDJIA
Messaouda OUDJEHIH

Healthcare-associated infectious risk management and medical simulation

Hanane BENALDJIA
Messaouda OUDJEHIH

Healthcare-associated infectious risk management and medical simulation

ScienciaScripts

Imprint
Any brand names and product names mentioned in this book are subject to trademark, brand or patent protection and are trademarks or registered trademarks of their respective holders. The use of brand names, product names, common names, trade names, product descriptions etc. even without a particular marking in this work is in no way to be construed to mean that such names may be regarded as unrestricted in respect of trademark and brand protection legislation and could thus be used by anyone.

Cover image: www.ingimage.com

This book is a translation from the original published under ISBN 978-620-3-45522-9.

Publisher:
Sciencia Scripts
is a trademark of
Dodo Books Indian Ocean Ltd. and OmniScriptum S.R.L publishing group

120 High Road, East Finchley, London, N2 9ED, United Kingdom
Str. Armeneasca 28/1, office 1, Chisinau MD-2012, Republic of Moldova, Europe
Printed at: see last page
ISBN: 978-620-6-08710-6

Table of contents

List of acronyms and abbreviations

AES   Blood Exposure Accident

CDE   Chambre Des Erreurs

CHU   University Hospital

CVP   Peripheral venous catheter

DAOM   Garbage-like waste

DAS   Healthcare waste

HIW   Waste from Healthcare Activities with Infectious Risks

DM   Medical Devices

ECDC   *European Centre for Disease Prevention and Control*

EIAS   Adverse events associated with care

EIG   Serious adverse events

ENEIS   National survey on adverse events associated with healthcare

PPE   Personal Protective Equipment

GDR   Risk Management

HAS   French Health Authority

HDM   Hand Hygiene

HH   Hospital Hygiene

IAS   Healthcare-associated infections

MSPRH   Ministry of Health, Population and Hospital Reform

WHO   World Health Organization

OPCT   Sharp objects

PED   Developing countries

PROPIAS   PROgramme national d'actions de Prévention des Infections Associées aux Soins (national program for the prevention of healthcare-associated infections)

PS	Standard precautions
RIAS	Risque Infectieux Associé aux Soins
SF2H	French Society of Hospital Hygiene
SHA	Solution Hydro Alcoolique

1. Introduction

The evolution of treatments, technologies and care models can have therapeutic effects, but also represent new threats to care safety. An adverse event associated with care (AEAS) is defined by France's Haute Autorité de Santé (HAS) as "an event or circumstance associated with care which could have resulted or has resulted in harm to a patient, and which it is hoped will not occur again" [1-3].

Serious adverse events (SAEs) associated with healthcare are events that are unfavorable for the patient, of a definite serious nature and associated with care provided during investigations, treatments or preventive actions [4].

In 1999, the U.S. Institute of Medicine declared that the American healthcare system "is not as safe as it should be". It estimated that "44,000 to 98,000 patients die each year in U.S. hospitals as a result of preventable medical error" [5, 6]. Other studies show that the incidence of adverse events in the healthcare system varies between 4% and 16%, and that the associated avoidability varies between 28% and 51% [7-10]. AEIAS include medication errors, risks associated with surgical and invasive procedures, and healthcare-associated infections (HCAI) [11].

A review of the literature carried out in 2020 found that HCAIs accounted for between 12.2% and 26.5% of all HAIs [12-14]. They represent a major problem for patient safety [15-20]. Every year, they affect hundreds of millions of patients worldwide. Out of every 100 hospitalized patients, at least 7 in high-income countries and 10 in low- and middle-income countries contract an HAI [16]. HCAIs are responsible for prolonged hospital stays, long-term disability, significant personal costs for patients and their families, additional financial burdens and loss of life [15].

Preventing them should be a priority for any facility committed to a quality approach, and concerns all the people and services involved in healthcare [16, 21, 22].

The curricula of the various healthcare professions are constantly evolving to incorporate their latest discoveries, while patient safety knowledge must keep pace with them, and health science students must be prepared to deliver safe care [17].

Within this framework, the World Health Organization's (WHO) Patient Safety Programme aims to implement patient safety as a subject to be integrated into the curricula of health sciences students worldwide [23].

Preventing the risk of healthcare-associated infection (RIAS) is fundamentally based on standard precautions (SP) in hospital hygiene (HH). SPs are measures designed to protect professionals and patients against the risk of infection. They must be applied to all patient care, whatever their infectious status [16, 24, 25]. The list of these precautions was updated in 2017 by the French Hospital Hygiene Society (SF2H). It includes the following precautions: hand hygiene (HDM), personal protective equipment (PPE), respiratory hygiene, prevention of accidents involving exposure to blood (AES) or any other biological fluid of human origin, excreta management and environmental management [24].

A number of studies have measured the positive impact of systematic implementation of SP on patients, caregivers, the environment and the facility [15, 16, 18, 26, 27]. Training healthcare professionals in HH is the cornerstone of all HCAI prevention and control programs.

The WHO's Patient Safety Education Guide lays the foundations for students to begin to understand and apply patient safety in the face of various risks, in all their professional activities [17].

In addition to conventional teaching methods such as lecturing, which are often used, other innovative training techniques that allow integration and creativity, and are adapted to the care functions, organization of care and work in healthcare establishments must be sought, such as the use of user-friendly technologies, *e-learning* and simulation [17, 28].

Simulation is a pedagogical method used for staff training and assessment, to meet 03 groups of pedagogical objectives: cognitive, psychomotor and affective [29, 30]. It is a pedagogical method of great interest, widely accepted and desired by both students and teachers [17, 28, 29, 31].

In adopting a risk management approach (RM), the HAS recommends simulation methods based on reflective practice and debriefing, which have a strong impact on the anchoring of knowledge and the acquisition of individual and collective safety reflexes [32]. In scenario-based training, the student is trapped by certain errors, which he or she is required to identify and correct in a context similar to reality - a "simulated environment". Alerted by these traps, the student learns and memorizes these simulated events better.

Simulation in the form of an "error room" (ERC) was first developed in Canada [33]. Several healthcare establishments around the world have drawn inspiration from this Canadian experience [33, 34]. The objectives of the CDE were to give warning signals by showing the pitfalls to be avoided, in order to reduce undesirable events and promote vigilance in the face of errors [29, 31, 35-38].

In recent years, in several countries, the use of this pedagogical technique in the healthcare field has developed both in the initial and continuing training of healthcare personnel [17, 32, 39, 40].

The ministries of health and the governments of these countries coordinate and promote collaboration on patient safety between and within sectors. Universities and health research institutes play an important role in this collaboration, by guaranteeing learning situations that promote training in the prevention of healthcare-associated risks, particularly infectious risks [23]. PS training in HH is an essential component of RIAS prevention.

In Algeria, in recent years there has been growing interest in developing training for the prevention of HCAIs. In this context, in 2015, the Ministry of Health, Population and Hospital Reform (MSPRH) drew up national guidelines for environmental hygiene in public and private healthcare establishments [41].

In Batna, HH training is integrated into the initial training program at :
-The Institut national de formation supérieure paramédicale (INFSPM) from the first year (HH module),
-Medical school: in 6th year of medicine (epidemiology module).

Continuing education at Batna University Hospital (CHU) is provided by the team from the Hospital Hygiene Unit of the Epidemiology and Preventive Medicine Department (SEMEP), using traditional training methods: lectures with Power Point support, on-site awareness-raising and display of protocols ...

Since the creation of the "Gestion du Risque Infectieux Associé aux Soins" (GRIAS) research laboratory in 2012, the SEMEP at CHU Batna has introduced MDM methods into its RIAS prevention approach as well as into training concerning this risk.

2. Adverse events associated with care

Zero risk does not exist in all human activities. Healthcare is a complex, highly technical system that involves human behavior, complex care organizations and the fragility of the patient.

With the scientific discoveries of modern medicine, the continuous evolution of new treatments and care technologies in healthcare systems can have satisfying therapeutic effects, but also represent new threats to care activities. Studies from many countries show that, as a result of these threats, patients can suffer damage that may leave permanent sequelae, prolong hospital stays or even lead to death [17, 23, 42, 43].

An AEIAS was defined in 2006 by the WHO as follows: "a patient safety incident is an event or circumstance that could have resulted, or has resulted, in unnecessary harm to a patient" [44]. The HAS has added "and which it is hoped will not occur again" to this definition [1-3]. HCAIs include: HCAIs, medication errors, risks associated with surgical and invasive procedures, etc. [11].

In 1999, the American Institute of Medicine declared that the American healthcare system "is not as safe as it should be". It published its report "*To err is human*", in which it estimated that "44,000 to 98,000 patients die each year in U.S. hospitals as a result of preventable medical error. These preventable errors cause more deaths than car accidents, breast cancer and AIDS combined" [6]. According to the systematic review by De Vries et al. of eight studies (74,485 patients), 9.2% of hospital admissions were due to an AEIAS [45]. Studies show that the incidence of AEIAS exceeds 10% in developed countries [11, 46]. They are caused by a variety of adverse events, up to 50% of which are preventable [45].

Patient harm caused by adverse events is one of the top 10 causes of death and disability worldwide [23]. Every year, 134 million adverse events due to unsafe care occur in hospitals in low- and middle-income countries, contributing to 2.5 million deaths [47].

According to another study, around two-thirds of the global burden of adverse events following unsafe care, including disability-adjusted life-years lost, occurs in low- and middle-income countries [48].

Investments to enhance patient safety can generate consistent savings and improve patient outcomes [46]. Estimates show that around one in 10 patients in high-income countries suffers harm while receiving care in hospital [49].

Available data suggests that, in the countries of the Organization for Economic Cooperation and Development (OECD), 15% of hospital expenditure and activity is attributable to the management of safety-related problems [46].

Poor-quality care costs $1.4 trillion to $1.6 trillion a year in lost productivity in low- and middle-income countries, while the cost of HCAIs in Europe is estimated at 13 to 24 billion euros/year, and in the United States at $6.5 billion in 2004 [11, 47].

2.1 Patient safety

2.1.1 Definitions

A hazard is defined as the potential for harm or nuisance to people, property or the environment. It can be a substance (toxic product...), an agent (virus...), a phenomenon (flood, earthquake...) or a process (diagnostic error, administrative error...) [50]. The WHO defines it as "a circumstance, an agent or an act that can lead to a risk or increase the probability of its occurrence" [51].

A risk is an uncertainty, threat or opportunity that the business needs to anticipate, understand and manage in order to protect its assets and value, and achieve the objectives defined as part of its strategy [52].

An error is the failure to carry out a planned action as intended (execution error), or the use of the wrong plan to achieve an objective (planning error). An error can be an act of commission or an act of omission [53].

Patient safety is the absence of exposure to danger and protection against the occurrence or risk of harm, and aims to reduce the risk of adverse events to an acceptable level [51].

2.1.2 The evolving concept of patient safety

In the fourth century B.C., Hippocrates laid the foundations of a medicine that incorporated patient safety into its philosophy and practice. With his Latin expression *"Primum non nocere"*, he defined the goal of medicine, i.e.: in the face of disease, we must have two things in mind: to do good, or at least to do no harm, not to harm the patient [54]. Since then, this phrase has been taught to all students of the healthcare professions. This phrase reminds healthcare professionals that all efforts to provide help must take into account potential adverse effects.

Centuries later, in 1847, Ignaz Philipp Semmelweis, an obstetrician, demonstrated the link between HDM and puerperal fever. He demonstrated that washing doctors' hands reduced deaths in women who had just given birth [55, 56]. Handwashing was not accepted or supported by the medical community until two decades later, when Pasteur, Koch and Lister published evidence of germ theory and antiseptic technique [55]. Today, studies continue to be published on how to teach and enforce handwashing among healthcare providers [57, 58].

However, it was the publication of the report entitled *"To err is human"* that marked a decisive turning point in the history of the healthcare safety movement. This report indelibly highlights the importance of human factors in the occurrence of HAIs. It shows that 70% of errors are the consequence of a dysfunction of the various factors involving human beings and the interactions they have with each other and with the environment [6]. The report also puts forward recommendations for building a culture of care safety. In particular, it recommends the implementation of safety standards, as well as MDM systems that will enable us to better understand and analyze the etiology of incidents, and to implement appropriate corrective measures.

Patient safety is an issue facing all healthcare systems [11, 47], as many medical practices and risks associated with healthcare pose problems in terms of patient safety [23]. This is a growing challenge for global public health. Governments must make patient safety a priority in health coverage policies and plans, and provide political support and resources to integrate the fundamental elements of patient safety into health systems and emergency care [23].

In punishment-based cultures, people are afraid to report safety incidents because they are afraid of being blamed, and they cannot learn from their mistakes [23]. So, the original concept of patient safety is based on 2 key points; the first is that it doesn't make sense to punish people for making mistakes, and the second is that we can reduce the number of errors by improving the system [59].

The need for attention to quality of care and patient safety was first expressed by the World Health Assembly in 2002 [60]. Since 2002, several Regional Committee resolutions have focused on improving patient safety, and WHO has played a crucial role in shaping global action on patient safety, providing leadership, setting priorities, bringing together experts, fostering collaboration, creating networks, publishing guidelines, facilitating change, building capacity and monitoring developments [23].

WHO's patient safety activities began with the creation of the World Alliance for Patient Safety in 2004. And in 2005, the WHO's first Global Patient Safety Challenge, with the theme "Cleaner care is safer care", aimed to reduce HCAIs, mainly by improving HDM. In 2008, the second challenge, with the theme "Safer surgery saves lives", aimed to take action to reduce the risks associated with surgery [23]. In 2011, WHO published "The WHO Patient Safety Education Guide, Multiprofessional Edition" to facilitate patient safety education in universities, health science student training institutions and healthcare facilities [17].

Since 2016, health ministers, high-level delegates, experts and representatives of international organizations have been advocating patient safety to political leaders. In 2018, it took place in Japan, the Tokyo Declaration on Patient Safety [23, 61].

WHO collaborates with key international partners and cooperates with several countries to improve patient safety. It has created the World Network for Patient Safety to bring together a range of actors and stakeholders [23].

In the digital age, the use of digital technologies to implement patient safety interventions, and to monitor and measure their impact, is becoming indispensable. These technologies can help support and strengthen essential elements of patient safety, including incident reporting and analysis for learning purposes, monitoring of patient safety interventions, training of healthcare professionals and collaboration with patients and families [23].

2.1.3   Analysis of error

A great deal of research into the relationship between human factors and medical errors has led to the development of models that provide a better understanding of the mechanisms by which accidents occur. Among all this research, James Reason's Swiss cheese model remains the most widely used (Figure 1) [62, 63].

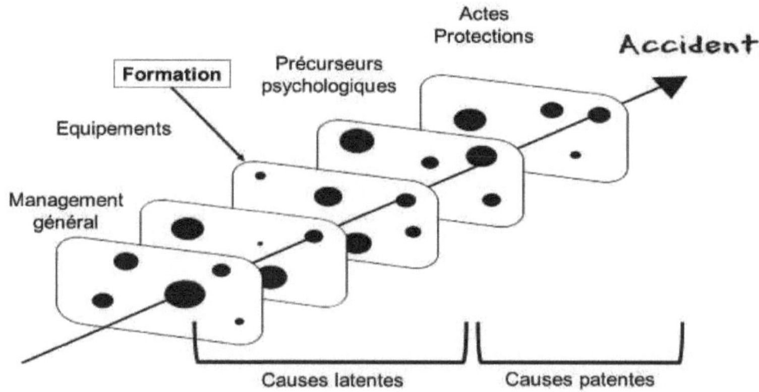

Figure 1: James REASON's Swiss Cheese model.

(Source: James Reason, "The Contribution of Latent Human Failures to the Breakdown of Complex Systems", *Philosophical Transactions of the Royal Society of London. Series B, Biological Sciences*, vol. 327, n° 1241, April 12 1990, pp. 475-484)

This model is a simple illustration of how patients suffer harm, based on a systems approach. In a complex healthcare system, errors are prevented by a series of barriers, defenses and protections represented by the slices of cheese. Each slice acts as a shield against failures. Ideally, all slices should remain intact, but each barrier has unexpected weaknesses or unstable holes that are constantly opening and closing, hence the similarity to Swiss cheese. If an error occurs and passes through the hole in a slice, this is not a major problem. There are usually no negative consequences. Sometimes, however, these holes line up across several slices, causing the defense system to break down [62-65].

When all the holes are momentarily aligned, patients are exposed to hazards and suffer damage. Two phenomena can explain these holes in the defenses: active failures and latent conditions.

2.1.3.1   Active failures (or patent conditions)

These are unsafe acts committed by people in direct contact with the patient. They have a direct and generally short-lived effect on the integrity of defenses. According to Reason [63], they manifest themselves in many ways:

a.   **Slippage** occurs when a plan is correctly established but poorly executed.

b.   **Failure**, when a step in the plan is omitted or forgotten.

c.   **Errors** are due to misinterpretations of appropriate rules.

d.   **Violation,** when a person is aware of the rules but doesn't follow them. Not with malicious intent, but to save time or complete a priority task.

2.1.3.2   Latent conditions

They are hidden in the design and operation of the system environment or equipment. They may lie dormant in the system until they combine with an active failure to create an opportunity for harm to occur [63]. They are responsible for weaknesses in defenses due to ineffective training, inadequate supervision, ineffective communication, inadequate staffing and long-term staffing [63].

The concept of MDM is not new, having been developed in the 1970s in the fields of insurance, security and finance, but it was in the late 1990s that its application exploded in the healthcare field [66].

In the hospital, patients are exposed to numerous iatrogenic risks. Every stage in the administration of care carries some risk for the patient, and adverse events can result from a hazardous environment in terms of layout or equipment, inappropriate use of equipment, misidentification of the patient, taking of inappropriate medical measures or lack of necessary measures, poorly performed procedures or failure to observe hygiene rules [67-69].

Improvements in patient safety require a complex system-wide effort. For example, the WHO has urged the introduction of measures to reduce iatrogenic risks [23].

2.2 Healthcare-associated infections (HAIs)

2.2.1 Definition of IAS

An infection is said to be associated with care if it occurs during or after a patient's care (diagnostic, therapeutic, palliative, preventive or educational), and if it was neither present nor incubating at the start of the care. When the infectious state at the start of care is not known precisely, a delay of at least 48 hours or a delay greater than the incubation period is commonly accepted to define a HCAI [70].

2.2.2 Epidemiology of IAS

According to the WHO, a significant proportion of all HAEs are represented by HCAIs, which are a major threat because they are responsible for significant morbidity, mortality and socio-economic burden for patients and their families [12, 71-76].

According to their anatomical sites, the most frequent are urinary tract infections, which account for 28.47%, followed by surgical site infections and pneumonia with 15.92% and 15.63% respectively [77].

These infections represent a universal public health problem [78, 79]. According to data from several countries, the prevalence of HAIs is around 7.6% in high-income countries and 10% in low- and middle-income countries [76, 80]. Several hundred million patients are affected by HAIs every year, and resistant infections cause at least 50,000 deaths a year in Europe and the USA [81].

HCAIs lead to longer hospital stays, permanent disability, high mortality and significant financial losses for healthcare systems and patients [82, 83].

In the United States, the incidence rate of HAIs was estimated at 4.5% in 2002, and around 100,000 deaths were attributed to these infections. The annual economic cost of HAIs was estimated at $6.5 billion in 2004 [84].

HCAIs are recognized as a major burden on patients, society and healthcare management. In 2008, the *European Centre for Disease Prevention and Control* (ECDC) estimated that over four million people contract a HCAI each year in the European Union, leading to an additional 25 million hospital days, with an economic burden of between 13 and 24 billion euros per year [84]. Around 37,000 people die as a direct result of HCAIs [85]. In England, over 100,000 cases of HCAI result in more than 5,000 deaths directly attributable to these infections every year [84].

In developing countries, the risk of HCAI is higher. Combined data from a limited number of hospital studies have shown that the prevalence of HCAI is15.5% [86]. A multicenter study carried out in 2003 to determine the prevalence rate of nosocomial infections in pilot hospitals in the Mediterranean region. The survey was carried out in 27 public and private establishments, including four in Algeria, six in Morocco and four in Tunisia, and the prevalence rate was 10.5%. However, the prevalence rates of nosocomial infections differ from one country to another: 7.9% in Algeria, 6.7% in Morocco and 13.2% in Tunisia [87].

In Algeria, a prevalence survey was carried out at the Bab El Oued University Hospital in Algiers to assess the extent of nosocomial infections. Among 426 hospitalized patients. A total of 69 patients were infected, representing a prevalence of 16.2% [88].

In Batna , the incidence of surgical site infections in neurosurgery at the CHU de Batna was 5.56%, 5.30% and 2.37% in 2014, 2015 and 2016 respectively [89].

This alarming trend has prompted healthcare professionals, managers, institutions and governments to pay more attention to the fight against HCAIs.

2.2.3   The fight against IAS

Preventing HCAIs is the responsibility of everyone - healthcare professionals, patients and administrators alike. Preventing these infections must always be a priority for all healthcare professionals, and therefore an essential element of patient safety programs [24, 25, 84]. A major consequence of the research carried out to better understand the dynamics of these infections, and to prevent and cure them, was the emergence of patient safety as a specialized discipline designed to help all players in a healthcare system to familiarize themselves with the concepts and principles of safety, and ultimately to prepare themselves to provide safe care [17, 90].

With the aim of managing HCAIs in hospitals, the concept of HH was born. HH is a discipline that involves implementing actions to prevent HCAIs and the spread of multi- or highly antibiotic-resistant bacteria, emerging or contagious infections [91]. The main preventive measures implemented to tackle this scourge are standard precautions (SP) [24, 25, 92].

In order to combat HCAI, strategies and methods are proposed within a legislative framework by Algerian regulatory texts. The first action was the creation of a national HH committee in 1998 by Ministerial Order N° 12 MSP of March 28 1998, whose role is to set up a program for the prevention of nosocomial infections [93], followed in November of the same year by the creation of a committee to combat nosocomial infections at the level of each health establishment, according to Ministerial Order N° 64 of November 17 1998, with the obligation to set it up [94]. This decree was followed three years later by Ministerial Instruction N°16/MSP/MIN/CAB of 20/10/2001 on the prevention and control of infections linked to medical practice. This instruction addressed the main issues relating to the management of infectious risks associated with medical practice, and set out the main recommendations [95].

These measures were followed by the publication of a number of regulatory texts focusing primarily on the management of healthcare waste (DAS) and AES. In 2015, the Ministry of Health's General Directorate for Prevention and Health Promotion published the "National guidelines for environmental hygiene in public and private healthcare establishments" [41] and in 2021 the "Guidelines for the prevention of infections associated with healthcare acts" [96].

At the CHU de Tizi-Ouzou, a study showed that after 9 years of implementing the recommendations of the Comité de lutte contre les infections nosocomiales, the prevalence rate of nosocomial infections fell from 12.06% in 2003 to 6.2% in 2012, further demonstrating that a return to hygiene measures is the key point in the fight against nosocomial infections [97].

2.2.4   Standard precautions in hospital hygiene (HH)

SPs are a set of measures designed to reduce the risk of cross-transmission of infectious agents between caregivers, patients and the environment, or through exposure to a biological product of human origin (blood, secretions, excreta, etc.) [25, 98]. They form the basis of the basic skills required in any HCAI prevention strategy, to guarantee the safety of care during patient management [25, 98]. They must be observed systematically: by all caregivers, in all care settings, for all patients, whatever their known or presumed infection status [24, 25, 41]. The list of these precautions was updated in 2017 by the French Hospital Hygiene Society. It includes the following precautions [24]:

2.2.4.1 Hand hygiene (HDM)

During treatment and prior to any HDM, forearms must be clear, nails short, without varnish, false nails or resin, and no jewelry (bracelet, ring, wedding ring, watch) must be worn [24, 25, 41].

Perform HDM according to the five WHO indications [99] :

1. Before contact with the patient,
2. Before an aseptic procedure,
3. After a risk of exposure to a biological product of human origin,
4. After contact with the patient,
5. After contact with the patient's environment.

Disinfection by friction with a hydroalcoholic solution (SHA) is the reference technique for all HDM indications in the absence of contraindications [24, 25, 41, 99].

2.2.4.2 Personal protective equipment (PPE)

PPE refers to the following barrier measures:

a. Wearing gloves

- Wear gloves only:

-When there is a risk of exposure to blood or any other biological product of human origin, and in the event of contact with injured mucous membranes or skin [24, 25].

-During care if the carer's hands contain skin lesions [25].

- Put on gloves just before the procedure; remove gloves and dispose of them immediately after the procedure is completed; change gloves: between two patients and for the same patient when moving from one procedure to another [24, 25].

b. Dress protection

- Wear a single-use impermeable apron or long-sleeved single-use impermeable gown when exposed to biological products of human origin [25].
- Apply protection just before the procedure, and remove it immediately at the end of a care sequence and between two patients [25].

c. Face protection

Wear a medical mask and safety goggles or a face shield if there is a risk of exposure to a biological product of human origin by spraying or aerosolizing. It is recommended not to reuse or reposition a single-use mask [25].

2.2.4.3 Respiratory hygiene

- Wearing an oral-nasal mask: medical masks (nursing masks, surgical masks) are designed to prevent the projection of droplets of saliva or respiratory secretions during exhalation from the caregiver to the patient, or from a contagious patient to those around him or her [25].

2.2.4.4 Prevention of accidents involving exposure to blood or any biological product of human origin

- For care using a perforating object: wear care gloves and use medical safety devices [25].
- After using perforating objects, do not recap, do not remove by hand.
- If single-use, dispose of immediately after use in a suitable sharps container as close as possible to the point of care [25].
- If the object is reusable: handle with care and clean and disinfect promptly.

- For treatments involving the risk of spraying or aerosolization, wear appropriate PPE.

The procedures to be followed in the event of an SEA must be formalized, kept up to date and accessible to all those involved in the care environment.

2.2.4.5 Excreta management

The risk of exposure to excreta arises mainly when handling excreta disposal equipment and during nursing care. Excreta disposal equipment includes various devices: bedpans, urinals, jars, commode buckets and pots in pediatrics [24].

Means of excreta management include bedpan washer-disinfectors, protective bags and grinders [24]. Manual procedures are to be avoided, due to the risk of exposure of professionals and contamination of the environment.

2.2.4.6 Environmental management

a. **Bionetting of surfaces and floors**: bionetting removes dirt and reduces biological contamination of floors and surfaces [24].

b. **Treatment of medical devices:** to prevent cross-transmission of microorganisms by reusable medical devices [24]. We distiguish :

Disinfection for heat-sensitive equipment.

Pressurized steam sterilization: this is the reference method for reusable medical devices, and can only be used for heat-resistant medical devices.

c. **Health-care waste (HCW) management:** The production of HCW must be subject to an elimination process adapted to each channel. Sorting waste at source is recommended, and must be adapted to the disposal channel and compliant with current regulations [24, 25, 41]. There are five disposal channels for SARs, distinguished by color code:

  - The yellow stream: corresponds to infectious healthcare waste (DASRI).
  - The red stream: corresponds to waste from healthcare activities involving chemical and toxic risks.
  - White waste: corresponds to radioactive healthcare waste.
  - The green sector: corresponds to anatomical waste.
  - The black channel: corresponds to waste that can be assimilated to household refuse.

d. **Linen management**: linen that comes into contact with the patient and is exposed to soiling by blood or any other biological product of human origin, must be disposed of as close as possible to the point of care, in a closed bag and through the appropriate channel, which must not be more than two-thirds full. Disposal should take place in carts strictly reserved for this purpose, fitted with a non-manual opening system and labelled to indicate their origin [24, 25, 41].

2.2.5   The benefits of patient safety training and HH

2.2.5.1   The benefits of patient safety training for healthcare students

It is imperative that everyone involved in care understands the extent of patient harm and why the healthcare sector needs to embrace a culture of safety [84]. Future healthcare professionals and health science students must also be prepared to deliver safe care.

While the curricula of the various healthcare professions are constantly evolving to incorporate the latest discoveries and new knowledge, the reinforcement of patient safety knowledge should feature on their syllabuses throughout the training and education of health science students. They should start applying patient safety skills and behaviors as soon as they enter a hospital, care center or health service [17].

Healthcare students need to know how systems affect the quality and safety of healthcare, and how to meet these challenges. The multi-professional edition of the WHO Patient Safety Education Guide lays the foundations to enable students, regardless of their chosen profession, to begin to understand and apply patient safety in all their professional activities [17].

Reason's Swiss cheese model [63], postulates that human errors, committed by individuals, only lead to damage in particular circumstances. These circumstances are latent failures, such as training failures. These latent failures can only be expressed through human action. To mitigate the consequences of these failures, measures are taken, constituting defenses in depth. Innovative tools such as simulation make it possible to act on an important aspect of latent errors, namely training [17, 100-102].

2.2.5.2   The need for HH training

HH training is an essential component of HCAI prevention and quality of care. It is the cornerstone of all HCAI prevention, control and patient safety programs. Compliance with SPs by healthcare professionals, including medical students, and the implementation of these measures are recognized as effective means of preventing and controlling HCAIs [103]. These measures protect not only the patient, but also healthcare workers and the environment [15, 16, 18, 26, 27, 79].

In developing countries, despite the effectiveness of these infection control practices, studies have shown very low compliance with these measures by professionals and students [104, 105]. The formative years are the appropriate time to acquire the necessary infection control knowledge and skills [103, 106].

HCAIs, patient safety and policy harmonization and related programs are the subject of increasing attention and activity [17, 107]. Infection prevention and control in hospitals began in the former Yugoslavia in the 1970s. HCAIs were supposed to be reported by doctors directly to public health institutes, but very few or no infections were reported [108].

Since the SARS epidemic, concerns have been raised about the training of healthcare workers in infection control. In Canada, a project has been developed to build consensus on a set of common core infection control competencies that apply to all healthcare workers [109].

The European Union has been promoting policies and interventions that harmonize the prevention and control of HCAIs in all member states. Its general policy is defined in the Council's recommendations of June 9, 2009, promoting training for healthcare staff in the prevention and control of HCAIs [110].

The European project "Improving Patient Safety in Europe" was launched in 2005, focusing on training in infection control and the epidemiology of HAIs [111, 112]. This project developed the "Core Curriculum for Infection Control Practitioners". In 2006, this project also explored existing HCAI courses in EU member states [111].

In 2009, the ECDC launched a project entitled "Infection control training needs assessment in the European Union", with the aim of strengthening HCAI and HH control training in EU member states [107]. On the other hand, obstacles to the harmonization and promotion of HH and infection control training have been identified, principally differences between countries, namely the qualifications required of healthcare professionals, the resources available and the sustainability of HCAI control programs [107].

In 2013, ECDC published core competencies for HH and infection control professionals in the European Union and launched a second project entitled "Infection control training in Europe - implementation strategy" aimed at implementing and harmonizing infection control and HH programs and tools [112].

The WHO Infection Prevention and Control Core Components assessment tools are based on the document published by WHO in 2017, entitled: "Core components of infection prevention and control programs" [113]. It contains 8 core components of infection prevention and control programs at healthcare facility level, which are essential for strengthening HCAI prevention capacity and preparing an effective response to emergency situations involving communicable diseases. The third component corresponds to the provision of infection prevention and control education for all caregivers through participatory strategies including bedside and simulation training [113].

In France, the fifth recommendation of the national technical committee on nosocomial infections [38] states that "initial training in HH is an essential prerequisite for all healthcare professionals working in a hospital establishment ... and the basic training of doctors is based on introductory courses in healthcare, on teaching in the first and second cycles of medical studies and on the internship program; HH must be integrated into the evaluation of clinical courses" [78, 114]. For medical students, awareness of HH is raised at the start of the second year of their studies, during the compulsory internship [24].

According to the findings of evaluations of the effectiveness of hospital-acquired infection control, it is important for hospitals to develop a continuous approach to HCAI control that includes: surveillance, the availability of specialized and properly trained staff, evidence-based policies and follow-up to ensure that recommended interventions are applied effectively [112, 115].

In this context, the initial training of health science students and the ongoing training of healthcare professionals in the fight against HCAIs are among the objectives and priorities of France's national program for the prevention of healthcare-associated infections (PROPIAS) [116], the WHO's patient safety program and other similar projects aimed at implementing patient safety worldwide [17].

But despite the available evidence, implementation of these measures remains a problem for both healthcare organizations and healthcare professionals, so it is essential to promote competency-based training in HCAI control among healthcare professionals in general, to raise awareness of the risks associated with HCAIs, their prevention and to make recommendations available to them [107, 117-119].

A variety of terms are used to describe "competencies", all of which relate to what the individual will know, understand and be able to do at the end of a learning experience. According to J. Tardif, a competence is: "a complex knowledge-action based on the effective mobilization and combination of a variety of internal and external resources within a family of situations" [120]. The term "basic skills" indicates that competencies should be a minimum prerequisite, common to all professionals in a field [107, 112].

Preventing HCAIs is part of a classic quality approach: identifying the risk, informing and training those involved, applying validated measures and evaluating their implementation. For this reason, it is essential that all healthcare professionals receive appropriate, regularly updated training in HH and the fight against HCAIs. Guaranteeing HH training for healthcare facility staff must therefore be an institutional priority [17, 121]. Initial and ongoing training in HH is no longer considered a luxury today, but rather a necessity, as it enables staff to acquire the practical and theoretical knowledge they need to continue to perform their duties properly, and to improve their skills in the light of dramatic technological and scientific developments and increased demands for improved quality of care [17, 121].

To be effective, HH training must use appropriate adult learning methods and resources. It must be adapted to the audience concerned, and in particular to the types of activities and missions of the personnel concerned [121].

The training provided must also be directly related to the tasks to be carried out by the staff to be trained. To guarantee maximum effectiveness, we prefer participative and interactive methods that place the learner in an active situation [121]. The aim is to get as close as possible to real-life working conditions, hence the importance of learning in a professional environment, using real or simulated situations [17, 121].

2.2.5.3 Pedagogical principles essential t o   teaching and learning about patient safety

Most errors are the consequence of a succession of facts and/or behaviors that lead to an accident. The key is no longer to find out who made a mistake, but to identify why and how the defense system failed, in order to prevent a mistake from happening again. We need to move towards a positive culture of error, which takes into account all the underlying factors involved in the occurrence of an adverse event, in order to achieve a global understanding. It is therefore essential to provide professionals with theoretical and, above all, practical training in these concepts.

The publication of the "*To err in human*" report was at the root of the patient safety movement, which has seen simulation e m e r g e   as a means of rectifying many of these concerns [6, 57].

For patient safety training to translate into safe practices with improved patient outcomes, it needs to be engaging for students. As with any learning process, one of the key challenges is to ensure the transfer of knowledge to the workplace. An ideal learning environment is one that is safe, supportive and stimulating [100].

Leclercq and Poumay [122], from the University of Liège, have proposed 8 learning m e t h o d s ,   called the *Learning Events Model*:

- By observation and imitation
- By receiving oral or written information from the instructor
- By exercising or putting into practice
- By exploration
- Through problem-solving or experimentation
- By creation or debate
- By reflecting on our own cognition and learning.

The superiority of practical methods over theoretical ones is widely accepted today [17]. The majority of studies have shown that theoretical training has little or limited impact on compliance with hygiene measures in hospitals. Practical training in gestures, techniques and methods is therefore essential. But it would be insufficient, even if it complemented theoretical training, if it were not based on training in "savoir être", i.e. attitudes [121].

To apply these types of teaching, which are often combined, there are different pedagogical methods. Dr. Chiniara, from the Université de Laval in Canada, describes them as environments for delivering instruction. These may include reading materials, oral presentations, computer-based techniques (*e-learning*) or simulation. The latter differs from the others in that it is interactive and imitates reality to some degree [123].

Students who are reassured and encouraged tend to be more receptive to learning, and are better prepared to participate actively in learning activities. Every opportunity should be taken to practice "active learning", i.e. t o involve learners meaningfully in the process, rather than having them merely be passive receivers of information [100], the following phrase sums up active learning well: "don't explain to students what you can show them, and don't show them what they can do for themselves" [84].

The choice of teaching methods should be based on pedagogical objectives, not on the appeal of novelty or technology.

3. Teaching HCAI prevention through simulation at santé

3.1.1   Definition

Healthcare simulation is defined in North America as: "the set of devices enabling all or part of a patient care procedure to be carried out in a reconstructed environment. This includes simulation mannequins, virtual reality, partial-task simulators and simulated patients. Hybrid simulators, combining several of the simulators mentioned above, are increasingly used" [124-126].

According to the HAS, healthcare simulation corresponds to "the use of equipment (such as a mannequin or procedural simulator), virtual reality or a standardized patient to reproduce healthcare situations or environments, with the aim of teaching diagnostic and therapeutic procedures and rehearsing processes, medical concepts or decision-making by a healthcare professional or team of professionals" [127].

In the space of just a few years, simulation has become an essential tool in the training of high-risk professions. It allows us to immerse ourselves in the real world, to reproduce a variety of situations, sometimes rare in the real world, and of course to learn technical gestures without taking the risk of making a real mistake. This principle is applied to all processes that can be piloted: nuclear, chemical, airplane, train, ship, subway and medical [30].

Healthcare simulation is an exciting field that combines new technologies, adult learning and clinical healthcare practices. It is an innovative, active teaching method based on experiential learning and reflective practice [32, 127].

There are three approaches linking MDM and simulation in healthcare [128, 129]; an "*a priori*" approach (simulation as a method of error prevention: training for beginner error prevention and to validate an organization or work environment), an "*a posteriori*" approach (from real error to simulation based on the use of feedback results following the reconstitution of scenarios after an SAE) and a patient communication approach (preparation for communication with the patient about SAEs that have occurred or the announcement of a damage).

3.1.2   The history of simulation

The first written history of healthcare simulators dates back to around 500 BC, in the Sushruta Samhita, a collection of medical texts discovered in Kucha, which described natural materials that could be transformed into surgical training equipment [130]. Our early ancestors simulated throwing spears at trees before hunting wild and dangerous animals. All training requires a certain level of simulated experience. The Romans were the first to train individual soldiers in sword fighting using the palus, against which the soldier would strike his sword. The individual soldier would then simulate specialized formations with his unit and section, to train against potential enemy tactics. This simulated training enabled Roman soldiers and their armies to acquire exemplary discipline [57, 131].

Since then, simulation users around the world have created thousands of tools to train healthcare professionals, including life-size bronze casts of acupuncture points in 1026, the birthing machine founded by Angélique Marguerite "Le Boursier du Coudray" in 1751 and the first auscultation simulator in 1864 [57, 131-135].

New and revolutionary technologies such as the airplane brought decisive military victories. The first simulated aircraft was used for aeronautical training in 1934 [57]. After multiple crashes in bad weather during domestic mail deliveries, the US *Army Air Corps* slowly began to adopt the *"Link Trainer"* [136]. The Second World War saw a massive increase in the use of *Link Trainers* [57].

The progress of aviation simulators continued with commercial flights after the Second World War. Airbus Senior Training Advisor Captain Jacques Drappier explained that when he first flyer in the 1960s, flight simulation was very basic, and at the time, older pilots resisted it because it wasn't very realistic [57]. However, later a new generation of pilots in the 1970s grasped the benefits of simulation and embraced its use to train for situations too risky or costly to be taught or experienced during actual flight [57].

Although the black box flight recorder was increasingly installed on commercial flights from the 1960s onwards, its usefulness has been questioned due to a potential invasion of privacy. On March 27, 1977, two aircraft collided on the runway at Tenerife, killing 583 people, making it the deadliest accident in aviation history. The effectiveness of the black box was proven after the two cockpit recorders demonstrated that poor communication practices were the cause of the accident. This led to the development of the CRM (Crew Resource Management) communication system, which would be learned and practiced by crews through simulation [57].

The airline industry has since become one of the safest in the world, with 2017 being the safest year in the history of air travel, during which 44 people died in commercial aircraft accidents worldwide [57]. At the same time, more than 250,000 patient deaths were attributed to medical errors in the United States alone [137]. Healthcare continues to learn from aviation, which was behind the regular evaluation of healthcare systems and the improvement of outcomes through simulation [57].

The Information Age introduced electronic engineering and advanced computer technology into all aspects of life, and laid the foundations for the healthcare simulation industry as we know it today. During the last century, several "simulation pioneers" of the information age had created electronic patient simulators [57].

In addition, a number of companies worldwide, such as *Gaumard, Simulab, Limbs & Things, Cardionics* and *Kyoto Kagaku*, have advanced medium- and low-fidelity task trainer technologies, enabling learners to focus on the specific clinical skills required for general and specialist care. These include arms for practicing infusion placement, torso models for auscultation... [57].

Audiovisual recording and debriefing systems are another technology essential to the success of healthcare simulation activities. These video analysis systems enable facilitators to review learners' actions. They allow full high-definition recording and live annotation to highlight good actions [57].

The first Canadian simulation center opened in Toronto in 1995, shortly after the first in the USA. There were half a dozen simulation centers by 1999, and over 60 by the 2009 census

[126, 138].

Many simulation centers are located in hospitals, while others are in training institutions [30, 126]. In some cases, the centers were dedicated solely to simulation research. These centers bring together healthcare professionals-researchers from all professions (doctors, nurses, occupational therapists, paramedics, dentists) and specialties (medical, surgical), with non-healthcare researchers from fundamental disciplines including education, psychology, evaluation, anthropology or sociology [126, 139] .

Today, simulation remains largely underutilized [140]. Although the use of simulation in healthcare continues to grow worldwide, those entering the field should bear in mind that healthcare simulation has not yet reached full maturity, but is still in an ascending phase of development [57, 141, 142]. According to Captain Drappier, "it took a generation of new pilots to understand the benefits of simulation training", and perhaps healthcare too must wait for those currently learning clinical practices through simulation to become clinical educators [57].

Simulation has become routine practice in the teaching of healthcare disciplines in North America [126, 143-145]. In France, simulation in healthcare has taken off in a remarkable way, and the HAS recommends it as a method of continuing professional development (CPD) [146-150]. In addition, this training and risk management method is a priority in the French National Patient Safety Plan (PNSP), in line 3 "Training, safety culture, support", action 4.3: "Make simulation, in its various forms, a priority method in initial and continuing training to advance safety" [149, 151].

With the aim of improving the training of future doctors and with the reform of medical studies, medical faculties in Algeria are beginning to introduce simulation into medical training. The first medical simulation center is at the Algiers Faculty of Medicine, which was set up in 2014. This was followed by the opening of other centers in other faculties: Mostaganem in 2016, Batna in December 2018...

3.1.3   Simulation techniques in healthcare

Simulation in healthcare encompasses several methods and techniques, which are summarized in Figure 2 [123, 152]. Depending on the objectives of training programs, several simulation techniques may be chosen or combined. This classification distinguishes so-called organic simulation from non-organic simulation, which is itself subdivided into electronic or synthetic, depending on whether or not computer-generated information plays a predominant role.

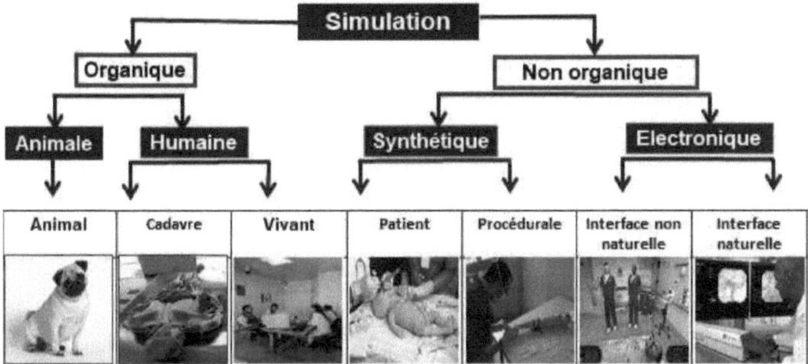

Figure 2: Different simulation techniques in healthcare (Chiniara, 2007)

(Adapted from: Chiniara, G. (2007) Simulation médicale pour acquisition des compétences en anesthésie. In: Société francaise d'anesthésie et de réanimation, Ed. 2007 Congrès national d'anesthésie et de réanimation, Conférences d'actualisation, SFAR, Paris, 41-49).

3.1.3.1　Organic simulation

a. **Animal experimentation:** used to practice basic surgical procedures such as suturing, or complex procedures such as laparoscopic surgery [30, 123].

b. **Human simulation:** this can take place on a living or dead human being.

- Cadaver simulation: one of the oldest simulation techniques in healthcare. Surgery, anesthesia and interventional radiology have described applications of cadaver simulation [30, 123].

- Simulation on a living human: using standardized patient or role-playing concepts.

  - ➢ The standardized patient (living human being): is a healthy person trained to simulate the history of a real patient and systematically reproduce clinical signs, personality, body language and emotional reactions. These techniques are particularly useful for training students in interpersonal skills such as medical questioning and physical examination, and for developing their communication skills [30, 32, 123].

  - ➢ Role-playing has lost none of its appeal in medicine, particularly for training in human relations and communication skills in crisis situations [30, 123].

3.1.3.2　Synthetic simulation

It is based on the use of mannequins that imitate all or part of the human body.

a. Procedural simulation: this allows training on a part of the human body by repeating technical gestures without risk to the patient. This type covers a wide range of procedures, often with a view to acquiring and mastering t h e gestures of a technique: intubation head, perfusion arm, etc. [30, 123]. Some simulators are more sophisticated and can reproduce highly technical interventional situations, such as coronary angiography simulators, complete laparoscopic surgery simulators, etc. [32].

b. Patient simulators: two main categories of mannequin exist, ranging from the low-fidelity mannequin (without computer) to the high-fidelity mannequin (computer interface controlled by an operator) [30, 123]. The mannequins follow a pre-established scenario; the trainer can vary their vital constants and clinical status, contextualizing them in an environment very close to reality [30, 32, 152].

3.1.3.3   Electronic simulation

a. **Natural interface (virtual reality):** combines computer technology and behavioral interfaces to simulate the behavior of 3D entities in a virtual world. It uses virtual reality headsets, for example, which superimpose virtual objects on what the wearer sees in real time [30, 123].

b. **Non-natural interface (3D environment and serious games):** uses simulation software consulted on screen interfaces. It is similar to the 3D environments found in video games, such as serious games [30, 32, 123, 152]. Their aim is to use digital game tools for a specific pedagogical purpose.

Some of these electronic simulation techniques can be very useful for EAD [152].

3.1.3.4   Hybrid simulation

This is a combination of several simulation techniques. For example, it combines a standardized patient with a part of a mannequin. This brings realism to the scenario by adding the patient's reactions [32, 123, 152].

3.1.4   A simulation session at health

A healthcare simulation session is typically organized in three stages: briefing, simulation and debriefing.

3.1.4.1   The briefing

This is a key stage in the session. It is essential, as it enables the learner to familiarize himself with the simulator to be used and the environment in which he will be operating [153]. During the briefing, the trainer explains to the learners how the session will be run and the instructions, and stresses the non-sanctioning nature of the simulation in order to create a climate of trust [30, 153, 154].

3.1.4.2   Setting the scene

After the briefing, it's the learners' turn to unfold the scenario, which can be guided by the trainer who adapts its evolution according to their reactions. The trainer's role and skills are essential both in constructing the scenario and in adapting it. The trainer needs to be familiar with the simulation-based teaching approach and the theme being addressed [30, 153, 154].

3.1.4.3 Debriefing

This is a very important part of the simulation session, lasting at least as long as the simulation itself. It usually comprises three phases: the descriptive phase, the analysis phase and the synthesis phase [30, 153, 155].

The descriptive phase is marked by the gathering of participants' feelings, and the trainer must establish a framework of trust so that everyone can express themselves freely, reminding them that no judgment will be passed [153, 155].

The analysis phase is often the longest. Its aim is to study situations where participants have shown inappropriate behavior. It allows us to really look in depth at what happened during the simulation session. It is during this phase that any errors that may have occurred are reviewed in detail, along with the reason(s) why they occurred. This phase should enable each participant to become aware of his or her strengths and weaknesses, and should always be carried out within a framework of free expression [153, 155].

The wrap-up phase concludes the simulation session with a reminder of the objectives and key points, enabling the learner to synthesize what has been seen. It is customary for the trainer to ask whether they could have done things differently, and how this simulation could have changed their way of doing things [153, 155].

At the end of the session, the learner can be given a document outlining areas for progress, the direction of future training, an assessment of what has been learned, etc. [30].

3.1.5 The limits of simulation in healthcare

Simulation-based teaching is being integrated into existing training programs in several countries [126, 156]. This integration faces a number of challenges:

- Financial cost: the main limitation is the considerable financial cost of setting up a simulation program. This is spread over premises, equipment and personnel [152].
- The presence of a qualified simulation trainer is essential for the development of train-the-trainer courses [126, 152, 157, 158].
- The emotional and stressful aspect that simulation can generate in learners. The briefing plays a key role in reassuring participants [153].
- The culture of teachers, accustomed first as students and then as trainers to traditional teaching techniques [126, 159].
- Integrating simulation into training courses is time-consuming for teachers, as it often requires teaching in small groups [30].

3.1.6   The benefits of simulation in healthcare

3.1.6.1   An active teaching method

It is an innovative, active teaching method based on experiential learning and reflective practice [153]. In the 1980s, David Kolb became interested in learning and learning styles. In his book *Experiential Learning* [160], he argues that learning is most effective and powerful when it is based on personal experience and, above all, when it is followed by reflection on that experience (debriefing). Kolb devised a learning cycle (Figure 3). This cycle includes simulation, active experimentation, reflection on action and conceptualization.

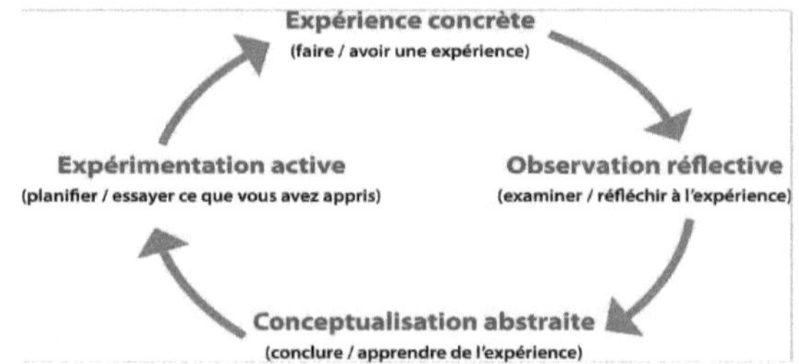

Figure 3: Kolb's experiential learning cycle

(Source: Kolb DA. Experiential learning: Experience as the source of learning and development : FT press; 2014.)

Simulation improves information retention, according to Edgar Dale's learning cone (Figure 4): after two weeks, we remember 10% of what we've read, 20% of what we've heard and 90% of what we've practiced [161].

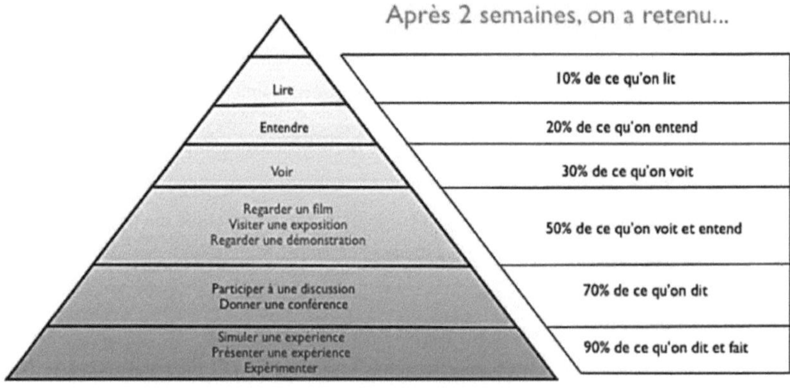

Figure 4: Edgar Dale's learning cone

(Adapted according to: Dale E. Audiovisual methods in teaching. Dryden Press, 1969. p. 748).

In this way, the learner can not only improve his or her knowledge, but also acquire know-how (technical gestures) and interpersonal skills (behaviors): numerous studies have effectively demonstrated the value of simulation in the acquisition of know-how [116, 162, 163]. Simulation is also useful for learning non-technical skills such as communication, leadership and team cohesion, where several studies have shown that learners feel they can communicate better with each other and work better as a team through simulation [32, 164, 165].

3.1.6.2   A guilt-free teaching method

Healthcare simulation does not punish error; on the contrary, it enables the professional to learn from his or her mistakes during the session, and particularly after the session during debriefing, through retrospective analysis of the various actions that took place, and awareness of improvement actions following learning. In addition, it is important to emphasize the importance of the trainer's supervision of the occurrence of errors, so as not to lead to a feeling of failure on the part of the learner, which could be non-pedagogical [127, 152].

3.1.6.3   An ethical teaching method

One of the main objectives of simulation in healthcare is to respect the ethical principle of "Never the first time on the patient" [30].

3.1.6.4   A method to ensure a sense of personal effectiveness

Simulation enables the learner to train in complete safety, both for the patient and for himself. This will enable them to make their practices safer and boost their self-confidence by developing their sense of self-efficacy [32, 152].

3.1.6.5   A recognized teaching method for training in healthcare risk management

HCAEs occurring in healthcare establishments are frequent but often avoidable. They are often secondary to shortcomings in organization, coordination, verification or communication, and therefore to a lack of a common safety culture [6].

In France, in the 2013-2017 national patient safety program, one of the operational objectives was to "Make simulation in healthcare in its various forms a priority method, in initial and continuing training, to advance safety." [151, 153]. Healthcare simulation has also been recognized by the HAS since 2011, as a method of continuing professional development [148] and as an innovative teaching method contributing to the management of risks associated with healthcare [127].

In addition, simulation-based training in healthcare has been shown to reduce costs, improve performance and reduce the risk of medical errors [57].

3.1.7   The uses of simulation

3.1.7.1   Training

- All types of knowledge are taught: technical gestures through repetition-based training [126, 166-168], non-technical skills such as attitudes to consultation [126, 169], communication, leadership and teamwork [30, 126, 170, 171].

- Initial and continuing training.

- Interprofessional and interdisciplinary training: is expanding rapidly [126, 172].

- Training for the introduction of new equipment or care techniques (in surgery, for example) is often provided using simulators.

3.1.7.2   Training assessment

- Formative evaluation: evaluations using simulation are most often formative. They can contribute to the precise identification of training needs [126, 172].

- Summative assessment: aims to "evaluate learning" and assess performance in order to give a score. Summative assessment is used as part of the major development of certification and recertification of healthcare professionals [173]. Assessment for certification is already in regular use for paramedics and other paramedical professions. Simulation has also been introduced for recertification in the medical professions, with a limited role for the validation of skills in the medical professions, but is increasingly integrated [126, 173, 174]. OSCEs (Objective Structured Clinical Examinations), introduced in 1975, are part of academic examination modalities, and serve as a support for student assessment [126, 172].

3.1.7.3   Research

Simulation is used either as an object or as a tool. Simulation was first used in medical education research, for example, to answer questions such as the cost-effectiveness of simulation-based teaching, the development of learning curves for technical gestures [126, 175], the learning of consultation [126, 169] or the comparison of several simulators [126, 176]. When considered as a tool, simulation is a substitute for the use of patients for studies in medical fields, such as airway management [126] or human factors [177], critical situation management for decision-making [177], or the impact of stress on caregivers [178], and is currently focused primarily on optimizing resources for simulation-based teaching [126, 170] and the use of simulation in interprofessional and multidisciplinary teaching [179, 180].

3.1.8 The Chamber of Errors (CDE)

3.1.8.1 The origins of the CRC

CDE simulation was first developed in Canada by the Canadian Patient Safety Institute, and appeared as the "Chamber of Horrors" during Patient Safety Week in 2006 [33, 181, 182].

This Canadian experience then inspired a CDE set up by the Centre Mutualiste de rééducation et de réadaptation Fonctionnelles de Kerpape in France, as part of Patient Safety Week in 2011 [33, 182, 183]. Since 2011, CDEs have also been set up in other healthcare establishments in France and around the world [31], [33, 34].

The CDE is now a widespread tool in English-speaking countries, where several hospitals regularly use it for medical and nursing students, as well as for junior doctors [67]. A number of scientific studies [22, 184-188] have come to positive conclusions about this tool, for example: Farnan et al. tested the CDE with medical students and junior doctors.

3.1.8.2 The benefits of CDE

a. It is an MDM method whose ultimate aim is to enable learners to analyze, understand and learn from the errors they have experienced, so as to avoid their recurrence in the care services. CDE is a fun and interesting tool, as the simulation of incidents, high-risk situations and clinical environments makes it possible to learn from one's mistakes, without endangering the patient [30, 31, 38, 183, 189-192].

b. It provides an opportunity t o address patient risk situations, acquire and update skills, analyze professional practices, reconstruct and understand undesirable events, and devise solutions for improvement. In this way, it generates interest in patient safety among all those involved in a healthcare facility [182].

c. It is part of the establishment's quality policy, which aims to encourage the reporting of undesirable events.

3.1.8.3 How the session unfolds

This is as realistic a patient room as possible. The room is set up like an ordinary room in an inpatient unit, but can also represent a specific environment such as a medication preparation room or recovery room, an operating theater, etc., in which errors on various themes such as hygiene, identity monitoring, medication circuit, hemovigilance, etc., are deliberately placed. [67].

As with any simulation session, it takes place in 3 phases: during the briefing, the trainer explains the pedagogical objectives of the session to the learners, who are invited to identify the errors, typically between 7 and 20, distributed at different points in the chamber. Following this exercise, which takes between 10 and 20 minutes, the learners are invited to debrief the errors with the trainers [67].

CDE is a tool appreciated by healthcare professionals. However, it comes up against a number of difficulties: logistical constraints (premises, equipment), human resources, limited access to hospital structures, difficulty in adapting errors to the target audience... [67]

This is a simulation using simple technical equipment to train observation skills, critical thinking and perception of the risks to which professionals and patients are exposed. Employees exercise their ability to identify acute risks. Unlike theoretical training, this method enables direct confrontation with concrete hazards in everyday clinical practice [67].

4. Assessing the lessons learned from prevention IAS

4.1.1 Definitions

4.1.1.1 Docimology: the word docimology comes from the Greek *"dokime"*, meaning

"Testing is the science of examinations. It aims to measure the quality of tests, in order to reduce the biases associated with the use of different assessment tools [193].

4.1.1.2 Evaluation: is defined by Nadeau as a value judgment made about a measure according to some criterion, with the aim of making a decision [194].

Evaluation is the process of gathering information about an activity or its outcome, leading to a judgment and a decision [195].

It is a continuous process that takes place throughout training, the modalities of which are ideally defined by teachers and their institutions. It provides *feedback* on student performance, teaching effectiveness and the quality of training programs and facilities [193].

For students of the health sciences, the aim of assessment is to attest to the ability of these future health professionals to make appropriate decisions and to act adequately to solve the problems they will face [193, 196]. This selection of competent professionals meets the need to protect society [193, 197].

Keith and Frese [198] focused on another possible impact of training: learning transfer. They found that training that encouraged people to make mistakes, as opposed to error-avoidance training, induced greater learning transfer.

Assessment has a strong influence on a student's motivation to learn, providing information that contributes to his or her sense of competence in relation to the proposed learning tasks. By helping them to perceive the value of these tasks and to identify the degree of control they have over them, it can foster student commitment and perseverance [195].

4.1.2 The objectives of evaluation

The objectives of student assessment in the health sciences are:

- Select candidates for a vocational stream or specialty.
- Certify skills acquired before moving on to the next stage of training.
- Certifying the skills of healthcare professionals to protect patients.

4.1.3 Types of assessment

How we assess determines how students learn. Therefore, in order to optimize and distribute their efforts, students will determine their working methods and the time they devote to learning according to their perceptions of teachers' expectations, the type of tests they will be subjected to and the possible consequences of assessment in the event of failure [193].

4.1.3.1 Depending on the moment of intervention in the training

a. **Diagnostic assessment (before or at the start of training):** This can be associated with two distinct objectives:

- Select students prior to training, e.g. in the context of a competitive examination, by identifying whether or not they have the ability to follow and pass a course [199].

- Measure students' initial level of knowledge at the start of their training, in particular by identifying any gaps in their knowledge [193].

b. **Formative assessment (during learning):** This is carried out on an ongoing basis and provides the student and teacher with objective information about a student's knowledge and skills at a given moment, with a view to adapting teaching and providing the necessary support as the student progresses. This formative assessment is non-sanctioning and leads the learner to intensify his or her efforts to identify strengths and correct shortcomings [195, 199].

c. **Summative assessment (at the end of the learning process):** This takes place at the end of a teaching sequence, to assess the degree and value of learning achieved by the student. It enables us to take stock of the knowledge and skills acquired by students, and any deviations from the expected level. It is "certificative" when it leads to the issue of a certificate, diploma or professional license. It is often carried out on the basis of quantitative assessment criteria, leading to the award of a grade [195, 199].

4.1.3.2 Depending on the nature of the assessment

a. **Normative evaluation:** when each student is evaluated in relation to the rest of the group, whose results are assumed to be distributed according to a Gaussian distribution allowing an average to be identified [195, 199].

b. Criterion-referenced **assessment:** when the student is assessed according to his or her deviation from one or more performance criteria [195, 199].

4.1.4 The assessment approach

Whatever the context and objectives, the learning assessment process consists of five stages: planning, data collection, data interpretation, judgment and decision-making [200-202].

4.1.4.1 Planning

Assessment is planned at the same time as teaching. The teacher selects the content deemed essential to the course and specifies the knowledge, skills and competencies that must be mastered. The teacher determines the target and the appropriate time for assessment.

4.1.4.2   Data collection

The decision to assess students and the choice of when to do so give rise to two further actions: choosing the type of data to collect and developing assessment tools.

4.1.4.3   Data interpretation

Interpretation concerns the teacher's reading of t h e assessment results obtained by the students.

4.1.4.4   The judgment

Judgment is "the central stage in the pedagogical evaluation process, which consists of giving an opinion on the progress or state of achievement of learning in the light of the various information gathered".

4.1.4.5   Decision-making

Following an assessment activity, the teacher must make a decision. Depending on the deficiencies identified, he or she may, for example, decide to return to the classroom, teach the deficient notion again, provide additional exercises, etc.

4.1.5   Choosing an assessment strategy

When choosing an assessment strategy, you need to think about the time you'll need to devote to the task, how assessment activities will fit in with learning activities, and which tools are best suited to the activity, since "learning" and "assessment" are closely intertwined.

With this in mind, it's vital to bear in mind that you won't be able to evaluate everything. Making choices will inevitably mean giving up some content and evaluation methods in favor of others.

To guide these choices, it is advisable to systematically seek coherence between the competencies expected of the future professional, the preferred teaching methods and the assessment strategies adopted. This coherence is referred to as pedagogical alignment [203]. Bloom's taxonomy [204] (figure 5) and Miller's pyramid (figure 6) are designed to help teachers achieve this alignment.

Depending on the underlying principles, if your aim is, for example, to develop (and thus assess) students' professional know-how, multiple-choice questions will be a poor assessment tool. If your aim is to have students acquire declarative knowledge, simulation will not be a relevant solution. The choice of assessment tools should therefore essentially be guided by the search for pedagogical alignment, in the knowledge that combining several tools is a way of optimizing the strengths and weaknesses of each tool [203, 205].

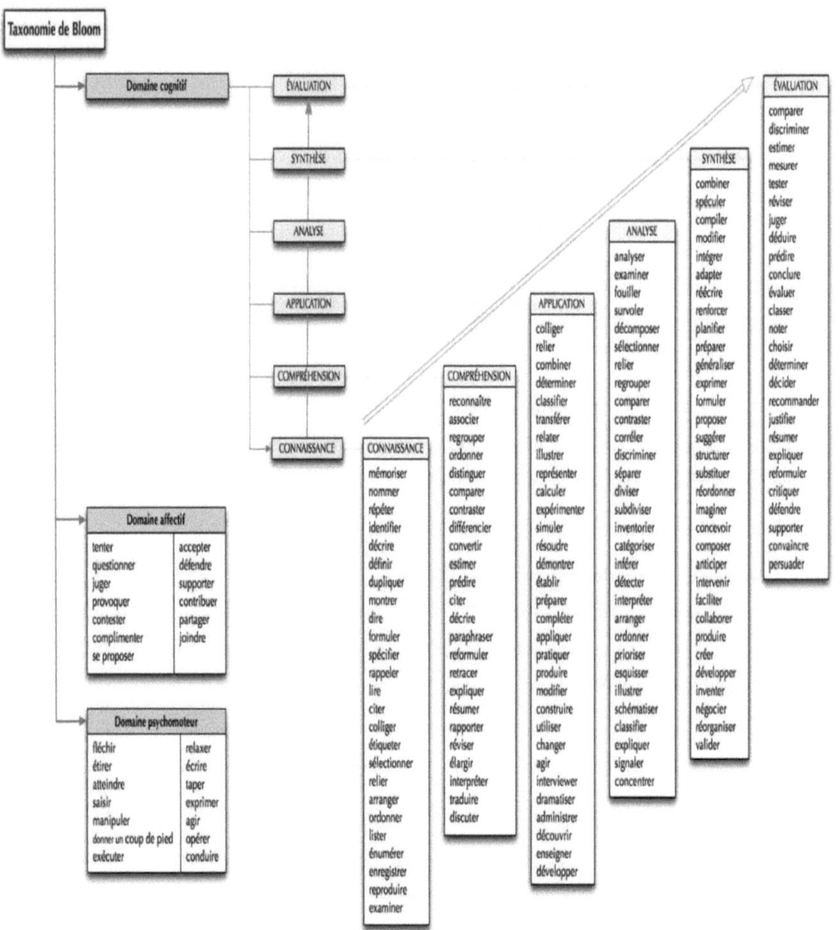

Figure 5: Bloom's taxonomy
(Adapted from: Bloom, Benjamin S., *et al.* Taxonomy of educational objectives. Vol. 1: Cognitive domain. *New York: McKay*, 1956, vol. 20, no. 24, p. 1).

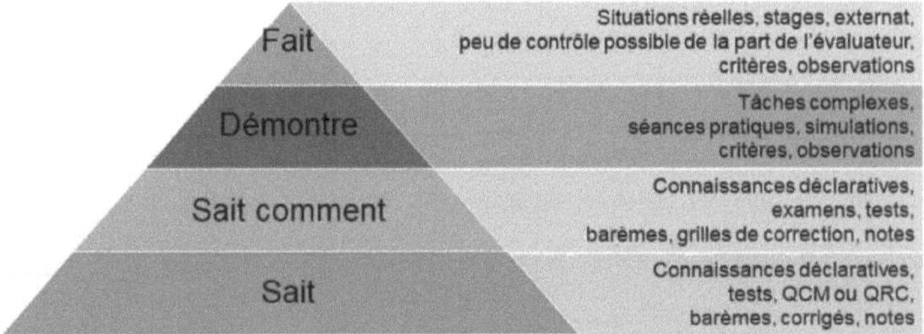

Figure 6: Miller pyramid

(Source: Miller, George E. The assessment of clinical skills/competence/performance. Academic medicine, 1990, vol. 65, no 9, p. S63-7)

4.1.6 The Kirckpatrick model

Kirckpatrick's (1959) four-level model of training impact has the advantage of synthesizing the complex process of training evaluation, and proposes a rational approach to meet the needs of training professionals (Figure 7). It is the model most widely used by training professionals, but also by researchers working on the evaluation of training actions, in order to assess several training objectives [197, 206-208]. It comprises four levels corresponding to complementary impact levels:

4.1.6.1 The first level

Called "reaction", it concerns participants' satisfaction with several aspects of the training (such as objectives, content, organization, teaching methods, materials, etc.). This is the level most frequently used [197, 208].

4.1.6.2 The second level

Measures participants' "learning" in terms of knowledge, skills and attitudes acquired during training. This is most often done by means of questionnaires or other systematized assessment systems (e.g. examinations) [197, 208]. Information is collected either by self-evaluation (level 2a) or measured (level 2b) [208], and some authors add level 2c, which corresponds to the knowledge and skills remaining after a given period of time following instruction [209].

4.1.6.3   The third level

Evaluates "behavioral changes" due to training in professional practice. This is measured by questionnaires or interviews to check that the knowledge and skills acquired during training are being applied in practice [197, 208].

4.1.6.4   The fourth level

This is the "results" level, which measures the impact of training on patient care, and the benefits to the patient [197, 208].

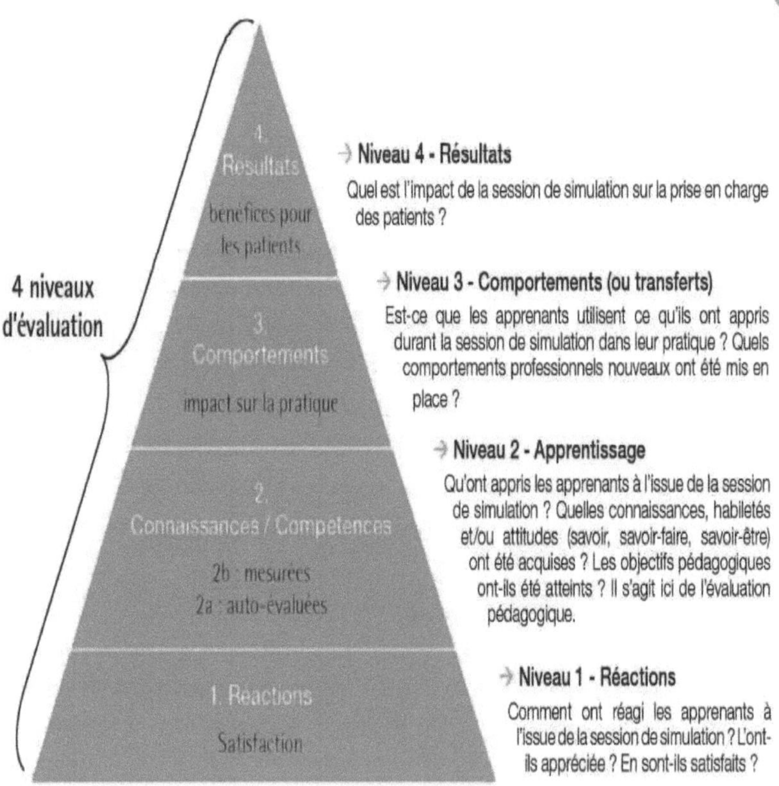

Figure 7: The Kirckpatrick pyramid

(Source: Kirkpatrick D, Kirkpatrick J. Evaluating training programs: The four levels: Berrett-Koehler Publishers; 2006).

4.1.7   Learning assessment at simulation

Simulation can be either an evaluation tool or a training tool to be evaluated. The evaluation of simulation programs concerns :

-Evaluation of the impact of the healthcare simulation session: this can be carried out using Kirkpatrick's model [208].

-Assessment of the quality of the infrastructure providing the simulation program, which must cover all its constituent elements: trainers, learner statistics, achievement of objectives, administrative organization, etc. [228].

5. References

1.   Haute autorité de santé. adverse events associated with care (AEAS). Patient safety - Managing risks. 2014.

2.   French Health Authority. Patient safety: HAS mobilizes to reduce risks associated with healthcare. Press kit Press office Saint-Denis La Plaine: HAS. 2015.

3.   Keriel-Gascou M, Brami J, Chanelière M, Haeringer-Cholet A, Larrieu C, Villebrun F, et al. What definition and taxonomy should be used for a collection of adverse events associated with primary care in France? Revue d'épidémiologie et de santé publique. 2014;62(1):41-52.

4.   DRESS. Les événements indésirables graves associés aux soins observés dans les établissements de santé : Résultats des enquêtes nationales menées en 2009 et 2004 (ENEIS). Solidar Santé. 2010;17:1-17.

5.   Homsted L. Institute of Medicine report: to err is human: building a safer health care system. The Florida Nurse. 2000;48(1):6.

6.   Donaldson MS, Corrigan, Janet M., Kohn, Linda T., et al. To Err is Human: Building a Safer Health System. In: Institute of Medicine Committee on Quality of Health Care in A, editor. To Err is Human: Building a Safer Health System. Washington (DC): National Academies Press (US); 2000.

7.   Thomas EJ, Studdert DM, Burstin HR, Orav EJ, Zeena T, Williams EJ, et al. Incidence and types of adverse events and negligent care in Utah and Colorado. Medical care. 2000;38:261-71.

8.   Magill SS, Edwards JR, Bamberg W, Beldavs ZG, Dumyati G, Kainer MA, et al. Multistate point- prevalence survey of health care-associated infections. The New England journal of medicine. 2014;370(13):1198-208.

9.   Baker GR, Norton PG, Flintoft V, Blais R, Brown A, Cox J, et al. The Canadian Adverse Events Study: the incidence of adverse events among hospital patients in Canada. CMAJ: Canadian Medical Association journal = journal de l'Association medicale canadienne. 2004;170(11):1678-86.

10.   Vincent C, Neale G, Woloshynowych M. Adverse events in British hospitals: preliminary retrospective record review. BMJ (Clinical research ed). 2001;322(7285):517-9.

11.   WHO. Module: What is patient safety? Course: the fundamentals of patient safety. 2015.

12.   Aranaz-Andrés JM, Aibar-Remón C, Vitaller-Murillo J, Ruiz-López P, Limón-Ramírez R, Terol- García E, et al. Incidence of adverse events related to health care in Spain: results of the Spanish National Study of Adverse Events. Journal of Epidemiology & Community Health. 2008;62(12):1022-9.

13.   Neal RD, Nafees S, Pasterfield D, Hood K, Hendry M, Gollins S, et al. Patient-reported measurement of time to diagnosis in cancer: development of the Cancer Symptom Interval Measure (C- SIM) and randomised controlled trial of method of delivery. BMC health services research. 2014;14(1):1- 10.

14.   Zanetti ACB, Gabriel CS, Dias BM, Bernardes A, Moura AA, Gabriel AB, et al. Assessment of the incidence and preventability of adverse events in hospitals: an integrative review. Rev Gaúcha Enferm. 2020;41(e20190364).

15.   WHO. Summary of WHO Recommendations for Hand Hygiene in Health Care. 2010.

16.   WHO. Prevention of Hospital-Acquired Infections: A Practical Guide. 2002;2nd edition.

17.   WHO. WHO educational guide to patient safety, multiprofessional edition. 2011.

18.   Hygis N. Hygiène hospitalière. 2010:57-66.

19.   RAISIN. Enquête Nationale de Prévalence des infections nosocomiales et des traitements anti- infectieux en établissement de santé (ENP) 2012. Institut de Veille Sanitaire (INVS). 2012.

20.   Fabry J, Carlet J. Controlling healthcare-associated infections: the first steps in patient safety. Médecine. 2016;12(1):36-7.

21.   Blumenthal D, Ganguli I. Patient safety: conversation to curriculum. New York Times. 2010:D6.

22.   Farnan JM, Gaffney S, Poston JT, Slawinski K, Cappaert M, Kamin B, et al. Patient safety room of horrors: a novel method to assess medical students and entering residents' ability to identify hazards of hospitalisation. BMJ quality & safety. 2016;25(3):153-8.

23.   WHO. Patient safety. Implementing healthcare risk management in healthcare settings From concepts to practice. December 11, 2018:1-9.

24.   SF2H. Updating standard precautions - Hygiènes - JUNE 2017;VOLUME XXV - N° HORS SÉRIE.

25.   CDC.   StandardPrecautions2018   .   Available from: https://www.cdc.gov/oralhealth/infectioncontrol/summary-infection-prevention-practices/standard- precautions.html.
26.   Hessels AJ LoE. Relationship between patient safety climate and standard precaution adherence: a systematic review of the literature. . J Hosp Infect 2016;4:349-62.
27.   Gammon J M-SH, Gould D.. A review of the evidence for suboptimal compliance of healthcare practitioners to standard/universal infection control precautions. J Clin Nurs. 2008;17:157-67.
28.   Vergnes H. Simulation in healthcare: a didactic and innovative teaching method for the prevention of infectious risk? [Professional Research Dissertation for the Master 2 in Education Sciences]2016.
29.   Granry J-C MM-CH. Rapport de mission - Etat de l "art (national et international) en matière de pratiques de simulation dans le domaine de la santé: Dans le cadre du développement professionnel continu (DPC) et de la prévention des risques associés aux soins. 2012.
30.   Boet S, Granry J-C, Savoldelli G. Simulation in healthcare From theory to practice: Springer; 2013.
31.   Yankova N. Safe administration of injectable drugs: evaluating the contribution of *e-learning* through an "error room" [Master in Pharmacy]: University of Geneva; 2015.
32.   Haute autorité de santé. Evaluation and improvement of practices - Guide de bonnes pratiques en matière de simulation en santé 2012.
33.   ARS OMEDIT Bretagne. Healthcare simulation tool: "La chambre des erreurs". 2013 Aug.
34.   Denry P. La " chambre des erreurs " : un outil ludique d "amélioration des pratiques, de la qualité et de la sécurité des soins Haute Autorité de Santé 27/02/2015.
35.   Doureradjam R, Dorsaz S. Simulation and training in nursing. Simulation in healthcare: From theory to practice. 2013:99.
36.   Vanpee D, Hosmans T. Simulation and technical skills. Simulation in healthcare: From theory to practice. 2013:141.
37.   Walker ST, Sevdalis N, McKay A, Lambden S, Gautama S, Aggarwal R, et al. Unannounced in situ simulations: integrating training and clinical practice. BMJ Qual Saf. 2013;22(6):453-8.
38.   Al-Elq AH. Simulation-based medical teaching and learning. Journal of family and Community Medicine. 2010;17(1):35.
39.   Alinier G. A typology of educationally focused medical simulation tools. Medical teacher. 2007;29(8):e243-e50.
40.   Lahti M, Hätönen H, Välimäki M. Impact of e-learning on nurses' and student nurses knowledge, skills, and satisfaction: a systematic review and meta-analysis. International journal of nursing studies. 2014;51(1):136-49.
41.   Expert committee for the prevention and control of healthcare-associated infections. Directives nationales relatives à l'hygiène de l'environnement dans les établissements de santé publics et privés. MSPRH. 2015.
42.   Brennan TA, Leape LL, Laird NM, Hebert L, Localio AR, Lawthers AG, et al. Incidence of adverse events and negligence in hospitalized patients: results of the Harvard Medical Practice Study I. New England journal of medicine. 1991;324(6):370-6.
43.   Leape LL. The preventability of medical injury. Human error in medicine: CRC Press; 2018. p. 13- 25.
44.   WHO. Conceptual framework for the international classification for patient safety version 1.1: final technical report January 2009. Geneva: World Health Organization; 2010.
45.   De Vries EN, Ramrattan MA, Smorenburg SM, Gouma DJ, Boermeester MA. The incidence and nature of in-hospital adverse events: a systematic review. BMJ Quality & Safety. 2008;17(3):216-23.
46.   Slawomirski L, Auraaen A, Klazinga NS. The economics of patient safety: Strengthening a value- based approach to reducing patient harm at national level. 2017.
47.   National Academies of Sciences Engineering Medicine. Crossing the Global Quality Chasm: Improving Health Care Worldwide. Washington, DC: The National Academies Press; 2018. 334 p.
48.   Jha AK, Larizgoitia I, Audera-Lopez C, Prasopa-Plaizier N, Waters H, Bates DW. The global burden of unsafe medical care: analytic modelling of observational studies. BMJ quality & safety. 2013;22(10):809-15.
49.   Slawomirski L, Auraaen A, Klazinga NS. The economics of patient safety. 2017.
50.   Desroches A. Risk management through global risk analysis. Clinical and biological

transfusion. 2013;20(2):198-210.

51.	Ceretti AM, du Lien F. Data on risks and adverse events related to care. Actualité et dossier en santé publique. 2012(79):23-46.

52.	Sghaier W, Hergon E, Desroches A. Global risk management. Clinical and biological transfusion. 2015;22(3):158-67.

53.	Balogh EP, Miller BT, Ball JR. Improving diagnosis in health care. 2015.

54.	Chaneliere M. Patient safety in primary care: conceptual framework, epidemiology, interventions with healthcare professionals: University of Lyon; 2017.

55.	Best M, Neuhauser D. Ignaz Semmelweis and the birth of infection control. BMJ Quality & Safety. 2004;13(3):233-4.

56.	Semmelweis IP, Murphy FP. Childbed fever. Reviews of Infectious Diseases. 1981:808-11.

57.	Baily LW. History of Simulation.	In: Comprehensive healthcare simulation: Operations, technology, and innovative practice: Springer; 2019.

58.	Pittet D, Boyce JM. Hand hygiene and patient care: pursuing the Semmelweis legacy. The Lancet Infectious Diseases. 2001;1:9-20.

59.	Leape LL. Error in Medicine. JAMA. 1994;272(23):1851-7.

60.	World Health Assembly. Quality of care: patient safety. World Health Organization. 2002.

61.	Third Global Ministerial Summit on Patient Safety. Tokyo Declaration on Patient Safety. Tokyo, Japan. 14 April 2018.

62.	Reason J. Human error: models and management. BMJ (Clinical research ed). 2000;320(7237):768- 70.

63.	Reason J, Hollnagel E, Paries J. Revisiting the Swiss cheese model of accidents. Journal of Clinical Engineering. 2006;27(4):110-5.

64.	Larouzée J, Guarnieri F, Besnard D. James Reason's model of human error: MINES ParisTech; 2014.

65.	Lederman R, Parkes C. Systems failure in hospitals-Using Reason's model to predict problems in a prescribing information system. Journal of medical systems. 2005;29(1):33-43.

66.	Bisaillon S. Risk management: utopia or stroke of genius? Pharmactuel. 2007;40.

67.	Chantal Zimmermann DLS. Interactive learning with an error chamber. User guide. 2019.

68.	Labelle V. Du travail du risque au travail institutionnel: la gestion des risques au quotidien dans le domaine de la santé: HEC Montréal; 2019.

69.	Benzidia S, Garidi S, Husson J. La standardisation des processus à l'épreuve des risques à l'hôpital. Management Avenir Sante. 2018(1):49-72.

70.	Comité technique des infections nosocomiales et des infections liées aux soins. Definition of healthcare-associated infections. Ministère de la santé de la jeunesse et des sports DGS/DHOS; 2007.

71.	Magill SS, Edwards JR, Bamberg W, Beldavs ZG, Dumyati G, Kainer MA, et al. Multistate point- prevalence survey of health care-associated infections. New England Journal of Medicine. 2014;370(13):1198-208.

72.	Zegers M, De Bruijne M, Wagner C, Hoonhout L, Waaijman R, Smits M, et al. Adverse events and potentially preventable deaths in Dutch hospitals: results of a retrospective patient record review study. BMJ Quality & Safety. 2009;18(4):297-302.

73.	Vincent C, Aylin P, Franklin BD, Holmes A, Iskander S, Jacklin A, et al. Is health care getting safer? BMJ (Clinical research ed). 2008;337.

74.	Pittet D. The Lowbury lecture: behaviour in infection control. Journal of hospital infection. 2004;58(1):1-13.

75.	Umscheid CA, Mitchell MD, Doshi JA, Agarwal R, Williams K, Brennan PJ. Estimating the proportion of healthcare-associated infections that are reasonably preventable and the related mortality and costs. Infection control and hospital epidemiology. 2011;32(2):101-14.

76.	World Health Organization. Report on the burden of endemic health care-associated infection worldwide. 2011.

77.	Santé Publique France. Enquête nationale de prévalence des infections nosocomiales et des traitements anti-infectieux en établissements de santé, May-June 2017. Santé Publique France: Saint Maurice, France. 2018:1-12.

78.	Comité technique national des infections nosocomiales. 100 recommandations pour la surveillance et la prévention des infections nosocomiales. Ministère de l'Emploi et de la Solidarité, Secrétariat d'Etat à la Santé et à l'action sociale. 1999.

79.	Nulens E, Gonzalo Bearman M, FSHEA F. Guide to infection control in the hospital.

International society for infectious diseases. 2018.
80. World Health Organization. Course: the fundamentals of patient safety. 2012.
81. World Health Organization. Antimicrobial resistance: Global burden. 2016.
82. Kakupa DK, Kalenga P, Baud M. Etude de la prévalence des infections nosocomiales et des facteurs associes dans les deux hôpitaux universitaires de Lubumbashi: cas des Cliniques Universitaires de Lubumbashi et l'Hôpital Janson Sendwe. Democratic Republic of Congo 2016.
83. Ouendo E-M, Saizonou J, Degbey C, Kakai C, Glel Y. Care-associated infectious risk management and service at the Hubert Koutoukou Maga National Hospital and University Center in Cotonou. Benin. 2015.
84. WHO. WHO educational guide to patient safety: multiprofessional edition. 2011. p. 17-31, 52-61, 211.
85. European Centre for Disease Prevention Control. Annual epidemiological report on communicable diseases in Europe: ECDC; 2008.
86. Allegranzi B, al e. Burden of endemic health careassociated infections in developing countries:

systematic review and meta-analysis. Lancet. 2011;377:228-41.
87. Amazian K, Rossello J, Castella A, Sekkat S, Terzaki S, Dhidah L, et al. Prevalence of nosocomial infections in 27 hospitals in the Mediterranean region. Eastern Mediterranean Health Journal. 2010;16(10).
88. Bezzaoucha A, Makhlouf E, Dekkar N, Lamdjadani N. Prevalence of nosocomial infections at the Bab El Oued-Alger university hospital. 1994.
89. Belkhiri F, Benaldjia H, Tobbi A. Gestion du risque infectieux lie aux infections du site operatoire au niveau du service de neurochirurgie, CHU-Batna 2014-2015. Dissertation for the diploma of special medical studies in epidemiology 2016:47.
90. Walton M. Teaching patient safety to clinicians and medical students. The clinical teacher. 2007;4(4):224-31.
91. DAGHFOUS HS. HISTORY OF HOSPITAL HYGIENE AND NOSOCOMIAL INFECTION CONTROL. HOSPITAL HYGIENE: Concepts, fields and methods. 2008:5.
92. ECN.PILLY. Infectious and tropical diseases.IAS2016. 937-8 p.
93. Arrêté n°12 du 28 Mars 1998 portant création du comité national d'hygiène hospitalière, (1998).
94. ARRETE N°64/MSP DU 17/11/1998 Portant création d'un comité de lutte contre les infections nosocomiales au niveau des établissements de santé, (1998).
95. MSP. Instruction N°16 /MSP /MIN / CAB sur la prévention, la lutte et l'éradication des infections liées à la pratique médicale. 2001.
96. Expert committee for the prevention and control of healthcare-associated infections. Guidelines for the prevention of healthcare-associated infections. MSPRH. 2021.
97. Prevalence survey of nosocomial infections. CHU de Tizi-Ouzou. 2013.
98. Southeast C. Précautions standard fiche technique. Coordination SSR Rhône réadaptation France 2011.
99. Safety WP, Organization WH. Implementation guide to the WHO multimodal strategy for hand hygiene promotion. Geneva: World Health Organization, 2010.
100. Davis B. Tools for teaching. JosseyBass Publishers San Francisco. 1993.
101. CCLIN. Principles of the ALARM-application method for infectious risk management. 2008.
102. Reason J. Understanding adverse events: human factors. Quality in health care. 1995;4(2):80-9.
103. Ayub A, Goyal A, Kotwal A, Kulkarni A, Kotwal A, Mahen A. Infection control practices in health care: Teaching and learning requirements of medical undergraduates. medical journal armed forces india. 2013;69(2):107-12.
104. Kotwal A, Taneja D. Health care workers and universal precautions: Perceptions and determinants of non-compliance. Indian Journal of Community Medicine. 2010;35(4):526-8.
105. Vaziri S, Najafi F, Miri F, Jalalvandi F, Almasi A. Practice of standard precautions among health care workers in a large teaching hospital. Indian journal of medical sciences. 2008;62(7):292-4.
106. García-Zapata MR-C, e Souza ACS, Guimarães JV, Tipple AFV, Prado MA, García-Zapata MTA. Standard precautions: knowledge and practice among nursing and medical students in a teaching hospital in Brazil. International Journal of Infection Control. 2010;6(1).
107. Brusaferro S, Arnoldo L, Cattani G, Fabbro E, Cookson B, Gallagher R, et al. Harmonizing

and supporting infection control training in Europe. Journal of Hospital Infection. 2015;89(4):351-6.

108.	Kalenic S, Budimir A. Education for healthcare associated infection prevention and control in Croatia: how to start from the beginning. International Journal of Infection Control. 2011;7(2).

109.	Henderson E. Infection Prevention and Control Core Competencies for Health Care Workers: A Consensus Document Compiled by: Dr. Elizabeth Henderson. 2006.

110.	European Council Recommendation. Council recommendations on patient safety, including the prevention and control of healthcare associated infections. 2009/C 151/01 of 9 June 2009 2009. Available from: https://ec.europa.eu/jrc/sites/jrcsh/files/2_June_2009%20patient%20safety.pdf.

111.	Improving Patient Safety in Europe. IPSE Consensus on Standards and Indicators. 2008.

112.	ECDC. Core competencies for infection control and hospital hygiene professionals in the European Union. 2013.

113.	World Health Organization. Guidelines on key components of infection prevention and control programs at national and acute care facility levels. 2017.

114.	Duroy E, Le Coutour X. Hospital hygiene and medical students. Medicine and infectious diseases. 2010;40(9):530-6.

115.	Haley RW, Culver DH, White JW, Morgan WM, Emori TG, Munn vP, et al. The efficacy oe infection surveillance and control programs in preventing nosocomial infections in us hospitals. American journal of epidemiology. 1985;121(2):182-205.

116.	L'Her E, Geeraerts T, Desclefs J, Benhamou D, Blanie A, Cerf C, et al. Interest of simulation-based learning in critical care. Joint recommendations from the Société de réanimation de langue française, the Société française d'anesthésie et de réanimation, the Société française de médecine d'urgence and the Société francophone de simulation en santé. 2019.

117.	Mathai E, Allegranzi B, Seto WH, Chraïti MN, Sax H, Larson E, et al. Educating healthcare workers to optimal hand hygiene practices: addressing the need. Infection. 2010;38(5):349-56.

118.	Pittet D, Allegranzi B, Storr J, Bagheri Nejad S, Dziekan G, Leotsakos A, et al. Infection control as a major World Health Organization priority for developing countries. J Hosp Infect. 2008;68(4):285-92.

119.	Wachter RM, Pronovost PJ. Balancing "no blame" with accountability in patient safety. The New England journal of medicine. 2009;361(14):1401-6.

120.	Tardif J. Conceptual reference points concerning the notion of competency, its development and evaluation. Organizing training around competencies A winning bet for learning in higher education. 2017:15-37.

121.	C ARFAOUI RH, B ZOUARI. HOSPITAL HYGIENE AND THE FIGHT AGAINST HEALTHCARE-ASSOCIATED INFECTIONS. 2008:85-7.

122.	Leclercq D, Poumay M. Le modèle des événements d'apprentissage-Enseignement. 2008.

123.	Chiniara G, Cole G, Brisbin K, Huffman D, Cragg B, Lamacchia M, et al. Simulation in healthcare: a taxonomy and a conceptual framework for instructional design and media selection. Medical teacher. 2013;35(8):e1380-e95.

124.	Girzadas Jr DV, Antonis MS, Zerth H, Lambert M, Clay L, Bose S, et al. Hybrid simulation combining a high fidelity scenario with a pelvic ultrasound task trainer enhances the training and evaluation of endovaginal ultrasound skills. Academic Emergency Medicine. 2009;16(5):429-35.

125.	Boet S, Collange O, Mahoudeau G, editors. Hybrid simulation: a new concept for new educational objectives. Annales francaises d'anesthesie et de reanimation; 2010.

126.	Boet S, Jaffrelot M, Naik VN, Brien S, Granry J-C, editors. Healthcare simulation in North America: current status and evolution after two decades. Annales françaises d'anesthésie et de réanimation; 2014: Elsevier.

127.	French health authority. Healthcare simulation and risk management. Tools for improving practices. Saint-Denis La Plaine: 2019.

128.	Moll M. La simulation la gestion des risques et la transfusion 5 eme colloque francophone de simulation en santé qualité et sécurité recherche pédagogique numérique. March 2016.

129.	Messarat-Haddouche Z. Health simulation and risk management project. Commission plénière des Pratiques et des Parcours. September 27, 2016.

130.	Champaneria MC, Workman AD, Gupta SC. Sushruta: father of plastic surgery. Annals of plastic surgery. 2014;73(1):2-7.

131.	Owen H. Early Examples of Simulation in Training and Healthcare. Simulation in Healthcare Education: An Extensive History. Cham: Springer International Publishing; 2016. p. 9-19.

132.   Gelbart NR. The king's midwife: a history and mystery of Madame du Coudray: Univ of California Press; 1998.

133.   Acton R. The evolving role of simulation in teaching surgery in undergraduate medical education. Surgical Clinics. 2015;95(4):739-50.

134.   Owen H. Simulation in healthcare education: an extensive history: Springer; 2016.

135.   Hureaux J, Urban T. Simulation in pulmonology: rationale, literature data and perspectives. Journal of Respiratory Diseases. 2016;33:A219.

136.   Page RL. Brief history of flight simulation. SimTecT 2000 proceedings. 2000:11-7.

137.   Makary MA, Daniel M. Medical error-the third leading cause of death in the US. BMJ (Clinical research ed). 2016;353.

138.   Hodges B. Advancing health care education and practice through research: The University of Toronto, Donald R. Wilson Centre for Research in Education. Academic Medicine. 2004;79(10):1003-6.

139.   Parker K, Shaver J, Hodges B. Intersections of creativity in the evaluation of the Wilson Centre Fellowship Programme. Medical education. 2010;44(11):1095-104.

140.   Levine AI, Schwartz AD, Bryson EO, DeMaria Jr S. Role of simulation in US physician licensure and certification. Mount Sinai Journal of Medicine: A Journal of Translational and Personalized Medicine. 2012;79(1):140-53.

141.   Gaba DM. The future vision of simulation in healthcare. Simulation in Healthcare. 2007;2(2):126- 35.

142.   Issenberg SB. The Scope of Simulation-based Healthcare Education. Simulation in Healthcare. 2006;1(4):203-8.

143.   Cooper S, Cant R, Porter J, Bogossian F, McKenna L, Brady S, et al. Simulation based learning in midwifery education: a systematic review. Women and Birth. 2012;25(2):64-78.

144.   McGaghie WC, Issenberg SB, Cohen MER, Barsuk JH, Wayne DB. Does simulation-based medical education with deliberate practice yield better results than traditional clinical education? A meta-analytic comparative review of the evidence. Academic medicine: journal of the Association of American Medical Colleges. 2011;86(6):706.

145.   O'Donnell JM, Goode Jr JS, Henker R, Kelsey S, Bircher NG, Peele P, et al. Effect of a simulation educational intervention on knowledge, attitude, and patient transfer skills: from the simulation laboratory to the clinical setting. Simulation in Healthcare. 2011;6(2):84-93.

146.   MOLL M-C, GRANRY J-C. Simulation: a factor in the development of professional skills. Risks & quality in the healthcare environment. 2014;11(1):21-5.

147.   Haute autorité de santé. Continuing professional development, Simulation in healthcare. 2012:6.

148.   Haute autorité de santé. Continuing professional development. Health simulation. 2019.

149.   Moll M, Granry J. La simulation: un facteur de développement des compétences professionnelles. Risques & Qualité. 2014;11(1):21-5.

150.   Granry J, Moll M. État de l'art (national et international) en matière de pratiques de simulation dans le domaine de la santé. Haute autorité de santé. 2012.

151.   Haute autorité de santé. National program for patient safety 2013- 2017. 2013:28 p.

152.   Colnot M. SIMERROR version 2. Evolutions and pedagogical deployment of a serious game on the chamber of errors. 2018.

153.   Haute autorité de santé. Guide de bonnes pratiques en matière de simulation en santé (2012). 2012.

154.   Jaffrelot M, Weiss A, Derrien P, Borraccia I, Vidailhet P. Preparing and running a simulation session. Pelaccia T, director How to (better) train and evaluate medical and health science students. 2016:249-68.

155.   Jaffrelot M, Pelaccia T. Simulation in healthcare: principles, tools, impacts and implications for teacher training. Recherche formation. 2016(2):17-30.

156.   Wilford A, Doyle TJ. Integrating simulation training into the nursing curriculum. British journal of nursing. 2006;15(17):926-30.

157.   Searle NS, Thibault GE, Greenberg SB. Faculty development for medical educators: current barriers and future directions. Academic Medicine. 2011;86(4):405-6.

158.   Sehgal NL, Sharpe BA, Auerbach AA, Wachter RM. Investing in the future: building an academic hospitalist faculty development program. Journal of hospital medicine. 2011;6(3):161-6.

159.   Savoldelli G, Boet S. Simulation session: from briefing to debriefing. Simulation in healthcare From theory to practice: Springer; 2013. p. 313-28.

160.   Kolb DA. Experiential learning: Experience as the source of learning and development: FT press; 2014.
161.   Molenda M. Cone of experience. Educational technology: An encyclopedia. 2003:161-5.
162.   Fiard G, Descotes J-L, Troccaz J. Simulation-based training: what tools do we have in urology? A systematic review of the literature. Progrès en Urologie. 2019;29(6):295-311.
163.   Shumard KM, Denney JM, Quinn K, Grandis AS, Whitecar PW, Bailey J, et al. Effectiveness of vaginal delivery simulation in novice trainees. Fam Med. 2016;48(9):696-702.
164.   Yee B, Naik VN, Joo HS, Savoldelli GL, Chung DY, Houston PL, et al. Nontechnical skills in anesthesia crisis management with repeated exposure to simulation-based education. The Journal of the American Society of Anesthesiologists. 2005;103(2):241-8.
165.   Garden A, Le Fevre D, Waddington H, Weller J. Debriefing after simulation-based non-technical skill training in healthcare: a systematic review of effective practice. Anaesthesia and Intensive Care. 2015;43(3):300-8.
166.   Friedman Z, You-Ten KE, Bould MD, Naik V. Teaching lifesaving procedures: the impact of model fidelity on acquisition and transfer of cricothyrotomy skills to performance on cadavers. Anesthesia and analgesia. 2008;107(5):1663-9.
167.   Barsuk JH, McGaghie WC, Cohen ER, Balachandran JS, Wayne DB. Use of simulation-based mastery learning to improve the quality of central venous catheter placement in a medical intensive care unit. Journal of hospital medicine: an official publication of the Society of Hospital Medicine. 2009;4(7):397-403.
168.   Boet S, Bould MD, Schaeffer R, Fischhof S, Stojeba N, Naik VN, et al. Learning fibreoptic intubation with a virtual computer program transfers to 'hands on' improvement. European Journal of Anaesthesiology| EJA. 2010;27(1):31-5.
169.   Bonnaud-Antignac A, Campion L, Pottier P, Supiot S. Videotaped simulated interviews to improve medical students' skills in disclosing a diagnosis of cancer. Psycho-oncology. 2010;19(9):975-81.
170.   Boet S, Bould MD, Bruppacher HR, Desjardins F, Chandra DB, Naik VN. Looking in the mirror: self-debriefing versus instructor debriefing for simulated crises. Critical Care Medicine. 2011;39(6):1377- 81.
171.   Jaffrelot M, Boet S, Di Cioccio A, Michinov E, Chiniara G. Simulation and crisis management. Réanimation. 2013;22(6):569-76.
172.   Reeves S. Ideas for the development of the interprofessional field. Journal of interprofessional care. 2010;24(3):217-9.
173.   Blew P, Muir JG, Naik VN. The evolving Royal College examination in anesthesiology. Canadian Journal of Anesthesia/Journal canadien d'anesthésie. 2010;57(9):804-10.
174.   Burwick RM, Schulkin J, Cooley SW, Janakiraman V, Norwitz ER, Robinson JN. Recent Trends in Continuing Medical Education Among Obstetrician-Gynecologists. Obstetrics & Gynecology. 2011;117(5):1060-4.
175.   Cohen ER, Feinglass J, Barsuk JH, Barnard C, O'Donnell A, McGaghie WC, et al. Cost savings from reduced catheter-related bloodstream infection after simulation-based education for residents in a medical intensive care unit. Simulation in healthcare. 2010;5(2):98-102.
176.   Friedman Z, Siddiqui N, Katznelson R, Devito I, Bould MD, Naik V. Clinical impact of epidural anesthesia simulation on short-and long-term learning curve: high-versus low-fidelity model training. Regional Anesthesia & Pain Medicine. 2009;34(3):229-32--32.
177.   Fioratou E, Flin R, Glavin R, Patey R. Beyond monitoring: distributed situation awareness in anaesthesia. British journal of anaesthesia. 2010;105(1):83-90.

178.   LeBlanc VR, MacDonald RD, McArthur B, King K, Lepine T. Paramedic performance in calculating drug dosages following stressful scenarios in a human patient simulator. Prehospital Emergency Care. 2005;9(4):439-44.
179.   Regehr G. It's NOT rocket science: rethinking our metaphors for research in health professions education. Medical education. 2010;44(1):31-9.
180.   Fincher R-ME, White CB, Huang G, Schwartzstein R. Toward hypothesis-driven medical education research: task force report from the Millennium Conference 2007 on educational research. Academic Medicine. 2010;85(5):821-8.
181.   Brifault C. "La chambre des erreurs" a healthcare simulation tool. CoClinnor CHU Hopitaux Rouen. november 20, 2015.
182.   Denis G, Legeas F, Chabosseau É, Gallien P, Nicolas B. The error room, to improve the quality and safety of care. 2015.

183.   Yankova N. Sécurité d'administration des médicaments injectables: évaluation de l'apport d'un e- learning au travers d'une " chambre des erreurs ", Master en Pharmacie.

184.   Trouiller P, Benhamou D. Room for errors in intensive care. Quality and safety in anesthesia-intensive care, MAPAR 2017. 2017.

185.   Teytaud M. Innovation pédagogique pour la manipulation aseptique à l'hôpital: développement d'un Serious Game: Université Toulouse III-Paul Sabatier; 2019.

186.   Joret-Descout P, Te Bonle F, Demange C, Bechet M, Da Costa M, Camus G, et al. The medication error room: simulating for better training. J Pharm Belg. 2015;97(2):10-9.

187.   Marry S, Cotteret-Couvé C, Loeuillet R, Videau M, Cisternino S, Schlatter J. Learning from mistakes: simulation of a centralized reconstitution unit for cytotoxic preparations. Le Pharmacien Hospitalier et Clinicien. 2019;54(1):101-2.

188.   Zimmermann C, Fridrich A, Schwappach D. Training Situational Awareness for Patient Safety in a Room of Horrors: An Evaluation of a Low-Fidelity Simulation Method. Journal of Patient Safety. 2020.

189.   Bruppacher HR, Alam SK, LeBlanc VR, Latter D, Naik VN, Savoldelli GL, et al. Simulation-based training improves physicians' performance in patient care in high-stakes clinical setting of cardiac surgery. The Journal of the American Society of Anesthesiologists. 2010;112(4):985-92.

190.   Doureradjam R, Dorsaz S. Simulation and training in nursing. Simulation in healthcare From theory to practice: Springer; 2013. p. 99-107.

191.   Vanpee D, Hosmans T. Simulation and technical skills. Simulation in healthcare From theory to practice: Springer; 2013. p. 141-50.

192.   Walker ST, Sevdalis N, McKay A, Lambden S, Gautama S, Aggarwal R, et al. Unannounced in situ simulations: integrating training and clinical practice. BMJ quality & safety. 2013;22(6):453-8.

193.   Pelaccia T. Comment (mieux) former et évaluer les étudiants en médecine et en sciences de la santé: De Boeck Supérieur; 2016.

194.   Nadeau M-A. Assessing learning in schools: a model for continuous assessment. Revue des sciences de l'éducation. 1978;4(2):205-21.

195.   Jouquan J. L'évaluation des apprentissages des étudiants en formation médicale initiale. Pédagogie médicale. 2002;3(1):38-52.

196.   Rosholm M, Nielsen HS, Dabalen A. Evaluation of training in African enterprises. Journal of Development Economics. 2007;84(1):310-29.

197.   Gilibert D, Gillet I. Training evaluation models: Individualistic and social approaches. PRATIQUES PSYCHOLOGIQUES. 2010;16(3):217-38.

198.   Keith N, Frese M. Self-regulation in error management training: emotion control and metacognition as mediators of performance effects. Journal of Applied Psychology. 2005;90(4):677.

199.   Bertrand C, Dory V, Pelaccia T, Charlin B, Hodges B. Understanding the general principles of assessment. How to [better] train and evaluate medical and health sciences students2016. p. 343-55.

200.   Loye N, Fontaine S. S'instrumenter pour évaluer. Pédagogie Médicale. 2018;19(2):95-107.

201.   Fontaine S, Loye N. L'évaluation des apprentissages: une démarche rigoureuse. Pédagogie Médicale. 2017;18(4):189-98.

202.   Leroux JL. L'évaluation des compétences au collégial un regard sur des pratiques évaluatives. 2010:83.

203.   Biggs J. Aligning teaching and assessing to course objectives. Teaching and learning in higher education: New trends and innovations. 2003;2(4):13-7.

204.   Bloom BS, Engelhart MD, Furst E, Hill WH, Krathwohl DR. Handbook I: cognitive domain. New York: David McKay. 1956.

205.   Van Der Vleuten CP, Schuwirth LW. Assessing professional competence: from methods to programmes. Medical education. 2005;39(3):309-17.

206.   Chiron B, Bromley S, Ros A, Savoldelli G. Evaluation of simulation training programs. Simulation in healthcare From theory to practice: Springer; 2013. p. 277-86.

207.   Bates R. A critical analysis of evaluation practice: the Kirkpatrick model and the principle of beneficence. Evaluation and program planning. 2004;27(3):341-7.

208.   Kirkpatrick D, Kirkpatrick J. Evaluating training programs: The four levels: Berrett-Koehler Publishers; 2006.

209.   Mosley C, Dewhurst C, Molloy S, Shaw BN. What is the impact of structured resuscitation training on healthcare practitioners, their clients and the wider service? A BEME systematic review: BEME Guide No. 20. medical teacher. 2012;34(6):e349-e85.

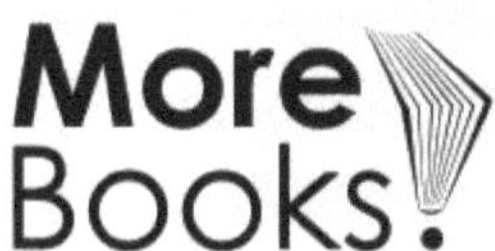

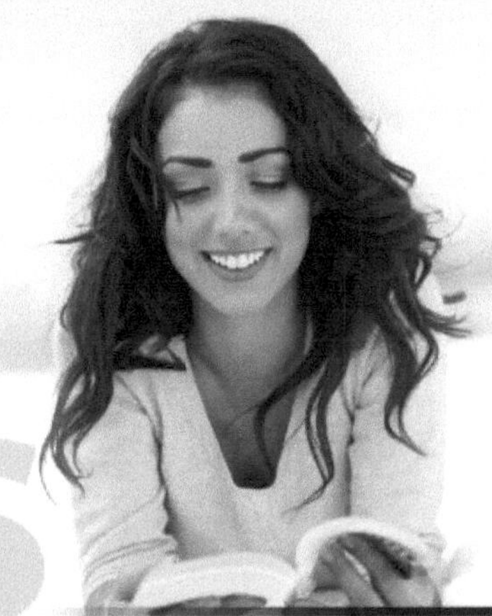

yes
I want morebooks!

Buy your books fast and straightforward online - at one of world's fastest growing online book stores! Environmentally sound due to Print-on-Demand technologies.

Buy your books online at
www.morebooks.shop

Kaufen Sie Ihre Bücher schnell und unkompliziert online – auf einer der am schnellsten wachsenden Buchhandelsplattformen weltweit! Dank Print-On-Demand umwelt- und ressourcenschonend produziert.

Bücher schneller online kaufen
www.morebooks.shop

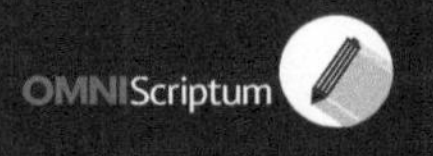

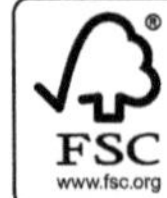